It's Not What We Bring,

BORDER
CROSSINGS

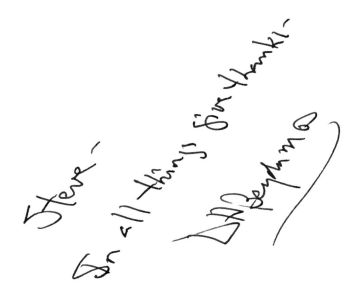

DAVID H. BEYDA, MD

Border Crossings
All Rights Reserved.
Copyright © 2016 David H. Beyda, MD
v1.0

Cover and Interior Photos © 2016 David H. Beyda, MD

The Holy Bible, New International Version, NIV, copyright 1973, 1978, 1984, 2011, Biblica, Inc. Used by permission of Zondervan.
New Living Translation (NLT), copyright 1996, 2004, 2007, 2013, Tyndale House Publishers, Carol Stream IL. Used by permission
The Jerusalem Bible, (JB) copyright 1996, Darton Longman & Todd Ltd and Doubleday and Company Ltd. Used by permission.
English Standard Version (ESV), copyright 2001, Crossway, a ministry of Good News Publishers. Used by permission.

Covenant Press

ISBN: 978-0-578-17910-0

PRINTED IN THE UNITED STATES OF AMERICA

*To all the children who are
brought into this world holding
onto life with one finger.*

"What you leave behind is not what is engraved in stone monuments, but what is woven into the lives of others."

Pericles (495-429 BCE), according to Thucydides

"Dedicate some of your life to others. Your dedication will not be a sacrifice. It will be an exhilarating experience because it is an intense effort applied toward a meaningful end."

Dr. Thomas Dooley III

(January 17. 1927 -January 18, 1961)

Acknowledgements

Sometimes I find myself looking around my world and seeing how many people have come into my life. There are many, some closer to me than others, some less involved and affective in my life than others, and some who are the foundation of my life. To all of them, I say thank you for being a part of my life.

There are some who do need some acknowledgment:

To the leadership of *One Child Matters* for their support and trust in our medical ministry. It is because of them that *Medical Mercy* was born and lived a decade serving 40,000 children in 15 countries.

To Kelly Ramsland, RN, my partner and co-founder of Medical Mercy. She was the backbone of coordination, the ever optimist that all would go well, even when we were faced with walls, burdens and setbacks. Her power driven faith gave me the fuel to trust in Him.

To all the regional directors, country directors, country medical directors, facilitators, project leaders, healthcare workers, teachers and cooks, who cared for the children in all the countries: you are the pillars of love and kindness for the children who came to you.

To the "core" volunteers who gave of their time to build Medical Mercy into a progressive and cutting edge medical missions organization: Darlene Schmerschneider for her IT skills, Micki Martin Pharm.D, for her direction and leadership in getting our medications in order, to Susan Ramsland for her skills as a pharmacy tech, and to Peggy Fullenkamp-Oomens, MS, RD, CNSC, for her guidance on nutritional support for those children who were malnourished.

To all the volunteers who traveled with us these past 11 years: over 180 of them, many making return trips of 3 to over 15 trips. Without you, we would not have been able to do what we did.

To Dwight and Kathy for your support and contributions in recognizing all of our volunteers. You have been a big part of Medical Mercy and its ministry and for that, many thanks.

To Bill Hammett, who when given a task to edit my words, took it on, made my words flow and gave them a polish that only Bill could have done. Many thanks Bill for all the hours of pouring over my blogs, taking the stories and getting them to read as one big adventure, and always keeping my words and style intact.

And to Charlcye, my wife of 35 years. You let me go where my heart pointed and where our God told me to go. You stayed home and cared for our family and made the trips I made possible by being the foundation of and for our family without question or frustration. You have given me more than I could ask for, and love everlasting. We are close to being able to enjoy our lives together as we step back from the world and focus on our sons, Nicholas and Justin, our daughter-in-law Rebecca, and our grandchildren, Nate and Molly.

Table of Contents

Foreword

As an editor, I get emails every day from people asking me to evaluate their books. I have to pass up most queries because there are just so many books I can take on in the space of a year, and most are poorly written or simply don't resonate with me. I therefore choose my projects carefully. When Dr. David Beyda emailed me, however, he told me that he was associated with Medical Mercy, which provided medical and spiritual care for his sponsorship organization called One Child Matters. He was, he wrote, overseeing care for 40,000 children in third world countries. He also sent a link to a blog he'd written over a nine-year period, noting that his one thousand followers were asking, "When is the book coming out?"

I clicked the link, and before I read the text, my eyes were drawn to pictures of people who had virtually nothing in the way of possessions. I saw a few smiles, but mostly I was looking at pain etched in the faces of the people David had photographed around the world. The faces were burned, misshapen, drooping, and scarred from accidents, abuse, and disease. All of the faces, taken together, were the face of the third world, and it was a portrait I hadn't seen before.

Then I began reading the text, which showed me places and a way of life that went far beyond the images I'd seen in television solicitations by various hunger relief agencies. The stories pulled me in, and I read about lives that had a raw, unfiltered essence that came through David's honest prose. The Forgotten Children, as he called them, lived in villages with names I'd never heard before because of their remote locations in the bush and various mountainous regions. They also lived in slums in large cities in Egypt and India, slums literally built with (and on top of) garbage. The words and photographs added up to a picture of dystopia, of people suffering in ways I hadn't imagined. Their government leaders—not that leadership was in evidence—were the "haves" and lived nearby behind their elegant palace walls just a few miles from the "have nots." At this point, I knew I would agree to edit the book because of the immediacy of David's words, words that brought me on his medical missions to Haiti, the Dominican Republic, India, Egypt, Swaziland, and Ethiopia.

But there was more. In *Border Crossings*—David had already chosen a title—I didn't just read about a doctor treating HIV/AIDS, tuberculosis, malnutrition, pneumonia, infections, cholera, and other diseases. I heard the voices of his patients, most of them children.

"I'm hungry."

"Can you help me die?"

"Will I ever walk again?"

"Do you know where my parents are?"

"Can you take care of my children? I have no money?"

I asked myself how such conditions could exist, even in third world countries. Where were the parents, the doctors, or the governments? I quickly learned that the children had been abandoned by their parents, political leaders, and by medicine itself in many cases. Hospitals were understaffed, illequipped, and even abandoned, although patients still showed up for treatment because of a sign on the building that said HOPSITAL (actual spelling).

As compelling and tragic as I found the narrative, everything I have alluded to thus far was only half the story. In our initial conversation, David was quick to point out that the story "is not about me." He was right. He wasn't after pats on the back or self-promotion as a savior who rescued the less fortunate. The book was about obeying God by serving His people, by ministering to the most wretched elements of humanity. David and his team, with great humility, were carrying out the mission of Christ to be His head, heart, and hands in the world, the Christ he had come to know in 1996 after years of struggling with the concept of faith.

In later years, he explained, that "concept" had become a dynamic, Spirit-filled way of living. Faith had come alive in a medical ministry centered on covenant relationships with patients. This ministry—this covenant—was about listening to God's call to serve the Forgotten Children, but not by merely dispensing pills in remote regions of squalor and hopelessness. This was care at its deepest level. Doctors and healthcare workers listened to patients, accepted them for who they were, and invested time in their spiritual welfare as well as their physical well-being. (The reader will be well-rewarded by reading Dr. Beyda's *Covenant Medicine: Being Present When Present*.)

Listening to God. Literally believing that He was directing people to travel to a specific country at a precise moment of time. Really? Was God still active in a world that seemed violent and lost, a world in which more than half the population goes to bed hungry each night? Those kinds of events happened in Biblical times, not the twenty-first century.

I had been a Christian since childhood, with a few lapsed periods along the way. I went to church and wrote an occasional check for charitable organizations, but that was about it. I prayed for the less fortunate, none of whom I would ever meet. Sure, I would edit the book. After all, David and I were on the same page.

But that wasn't entirely true, for as I immersed myself in David's eleven-year odyssey, I realized that many new pages were being added to my own book. The more I read, the more I knew that I'd been too smug in my posture as a caring Christian. The truth was that I had never seen poverty and suffering in such a vivid way, at least not since my youth, when "the cause" was everything in an age of activism. I also learned that I was not nearly as thankful for what I had as people in third world countries, who were grateful for waking up in the morning, clean water, and a single meal at noon. I had everything, and they had nothing, but they were the ones who valued gifts from God at a level of gratitude that shamed me.

But there was hope in the account I was reading. I saw that the Holy Spirit was indeed working wonders around the world, and that David had crossed not just national borders, but a border that separated secular concerns—a contract for mere technical services—from spiritual concerns and an all-inclusive relationship with "the other." *Border Crossings* rekindled a fire within me, enabling me to see that God is active in the lives of doctors, healthcare workers, pastors, businessmen, construction workers, and people from all walks of life—even a book editor who thought he had finally figured out most of life.

That's what I like most about David, who I now regard as a friend and brother in Christ: in the book he returns frequently to the fact that he doesn't have everything figured out. There is a lot of tragedy in *Border Crossings*, and it weighs heavily on his mind even though he and his team nevertheless continue their work, acting in God's name and not their own. They feed the hungry, care for the sick, clothe the naked, and offer hope to those imprisoned by despair.

I knew that missionaries existed, both medical and spiritual, but I'd never read a first-person account of what it was like to travel halfway around the world and set up clinics to examine hundreds of patients every day. And I'd never really seen the individuals who were hungry, sick, and dying. The details of their lives had been hidden from me until I read *Border Crossings*. In a journey of faith and obedience to God, Dr. David Beyda has revealed the stories beneath the stories, the reality beneath headlines of poverty, disease, and natural disasters.

Living this kind of faith can be a challenge. When Moses asked God for His name in the Old Testament, a voice from the burning bush offered a curious response: I am. I suspect that was a hard answer to ponder by virtue of its sheer simplicity. But voices also speak in the pages of *Border Crossings*. Some are very human, but perhaps there is a greater voice in these accounts, the voice of one who seeks to redeem all mankind. The children themselves will most certainly speak as you read their stories and look at their faces. As they shed their forgotten, invisible status, they will say, "I'm here. I'm alive. I'm real."

They, too, will say, "I am."

William Hammett
November 21, 2015

Chapter One

In the Beginning

It was disturbing, so much so that for a moment I thought I was going to pass out. The man lay there, unconscious, a crowd surrounding him and not sure what to do. The lion that had mauled him lay off to the side, dead. My father and I were out hunting when we saw the large crowd gathering in the distance, which was unusual since there were not many people living in the bush. But Somali warriors and village tribesmen can come together fairly quickly, either to do battle or to help each other. This was for the latter.

My father drove the Land Rover close to the crowd and got out, telling me to stay inside the truck. I saw the dead lion, opened the door, and stepped out, not wanting to miss what was going on. My father entered the crowd and quickly backed out, but it was too late to stop me. I was already there, making my way through Somali tribesmen leaning on their long walking sticks, chattering as they circled their fallen comrade. I reached the inner circle and saw a man on the ground. Bleeding, his flesh was torn and he wasn't moving. No one stirred or dared go near him. The tribesmen had speared the lion preparing to feast on the fallen man and now were wondering what to do next.

My father grabbed my arm and pulled me back, angry that

I had left the Land Rover, but I broke free from his grip. The tribesmen looked on and stopped talking as I moved closer to the fallen man, knelt down, and touched his hand. His finger moved and curled around mine. I looked up at the tribesmen and my father and then cried out "He's alive!" Oddly, nobody moved. The man's eyes opened and looked at me, and he slowly moved his lips. I leaned down to listen, inclining my ear to his mouth. He spoke one word: "Mahadsanid," which was "Thank you" in Somali. He never spoke again. I was eleven years old the day the tribesman died with a single word of gratitude on his lips.

"Why did you get out of the truck when I told you to stay put?" my father asked, the tone of his voice one that I realized was going to get worse.

"I needed to see what was going on," I said, daring to talk back even though I knew better.

"And what did you think?" he asked with a hint of unexpected gentleness in his voice. "Not very pleasant, was it."

"No, not very pleasant, but why didn't anybody try to help him? He was alive! No one even made a move to get near him. Not even you!"

"There was nothing to be done, David. He was dying. Unfortunate." My father had a thick accent, having been born in Egypt and later emigrating to the United States.

I was struck by the stark contrast between the two single words: "mahadsanid" and "unfortunate." One expressed thanksgiving, the other casual regret. They represented two very different ways of viewing the man's death.

"There *was* something to be done!" I said, looking at him with tears in my eyes. "In fact, there was a lot to be done: to simply *be* with him."

My father was silent while I cried as we sat in the Land

Rover. The Somali warriors were wrapping up their dead comrade and preparing to take him back to their village. Another group of Somali warriors was tying the lion to a pole to carry it back to the village as well, and I had lived in Africa long enough by then—it was August of 1962—to know why. The lion would be shown to the dead man's family, and the villagers would spear its carcass until all were satisfied that the man's honor had been made known. I'd seen it before, this spearing of a dead animal that had maimed a human. It haunted me, not because of the grossness of the act, but because of the futility of it. For whose benefit was it performed?

I was becoming accustomed to the established rituals to defend a warrior's honor—acts of respect for a man that were shown from a distance. Perhaps it would have been better if they honored the man by being with him as he died, praising him for his bravery and holding his hand. Wouldn't it have accomplished infinitely more than jabbing the lifeless lion? It was this very thought that set the tone for where I would be and what I'd be doing many years later: holding the hands of patients, respecting them for their courage, and honoring a covenant relationship between physician and patient, whether in the United States or crossing borders into underprivileged countries.

Born in Syria, my parents were raised in Cairo, Egypt. My father was college-educated, with a degree in mathematics, but he had a particular knack for languages, speaking seven in all. It was that gift that resulted in his tenure with the Foreign Service.

My parents emigrated to the United States in 1950, landing in New York City, where they found work in a clothing store. Not wanting to spend his entire life there, my father sought employment at the United Nations, thinking that his gift for languages would stand out. He immediately got a job as a simultaneous interpreter for the UN General Assembly. Using headphones, he talked to the diplomats who sat around the assembly table, but he wasn't there for long. The UN recognized his demeanor and his ability for diplomacy and transferred him to the UN Foreign Service, sending him to Somalia as a UN representative. I was five years old at the time. My parents were in the process of getting a divorce, and I was beginning to wander within the loose boundaries of an unstable family life.

My mother took my younger sister and me to Toronto for the next two years. I vividly remember looking up at the sky every time I heard an airplane flying overhead, wondering where it was going and thinking how much I wanted to be on it. It was then that I knew I wanted to travel. My father had sent me pictures of the African bush, of him in Mogadishu, and I was fascinated with the colors of the clothing that the Somali women wore, the fierceness of the Somali men—the warriors—and the general beauty of Africa.

In 1958, my father returned to the United States still in the UN Foreign Service, a status that was about to change. While in Somalia, the U.S. State Department convinced him to leave the UN and return to Somalia as a representative of the United States government. He made a quick trip to Toronto, where we met and talked. As the story goes, a week later I left my mother and met my father in Washington D.C. We left for Somalia soon after, and I didn't hear from my mother again until I was eleven years old. To her credit, she later told me that she knew I would have a better life with my father and become who I was meant to be. She gave up a part of her heart for me.

My father never remarried, and we traveled the world, moving from country to country. He was fully entrenched as a U.S. Foreign Service officer working for USAID, the United States Agency for International Development. In Somalia, I was looked after by two people who became my "family": our cook Mahmoud and our houseboy Mohammed. They cared for me like I was their own. They taught me to hunt, to speak a little of the language, to understand the cultures of the different tribes who lived around us, and to be observant. We would sit in a village to watch the routines of Somali life, and Mahmoud would ask me to tell him what I saw. At first I rendered basic, elementary observations: there's a camel, there's a mother with her children, and so forth. As time progressed, he taught me to observe more carefully and describe the characteristics of a camel, as well as the actions and movements of a mother, the children, and how they behaved. We also did this in the bush, observing the animals and how they grazed, hunted, and interacted with each other. He taught me that I had to first look for details before I could see more clearly, recognizing nuances of behavior that most people miss.

Now years later, I can spend hours observing people and get a fairly good idea of who they are. It has served me well as a physician since a diagnosis often entails more than a list of textbook symptoms. I really believe it was around this time in Somalia that I started to formulate the concept of relationships, the "contract" versus the "covenant." This covenant wasn't just about taking care of people; it entailed caring *about* and *for* them.

I learned to be independent quite early and made my first long-distance international trip when I was eleven, traveling to three different countries, staying in hotels, and getting to and from airports on my own. It certainly helped to have a diplomatic passport, and I was always greeted by a U.S. embassy representative and given assistance as needed when I arrived in a city. Although I was only eleven, I was far beyond the maturity of my peers and began to understand what I wanted to do for the rest of my life: practice medicine and take care of the sick in third world countries.

So how did the border crossings start?

Somalia wasn't what I expected, but then again I really didn't know what to expect upon arrival. The door of the DC-7 opened and a wave of hot air burst through, bringing with it the first taste of the Somali heat. Mogadishu was going to be the first of many places I would travel to and the one place that gave me the heart to live in or visit underdeveloped countries. On the horn of Africa on the east side of the continent, it rested next to the Indian Ocean and was bordered by Ethiopia and Kenya. It lay on the equator, giving rise to heat that would surround me for five years. I was seven years old, and the year was 1958. My father was stationed in Mogadishu, and it was there that I came to know the world of diplomacy, foreign aid, politics, and the underlying complexities of the third world.

In actuality, there was never a time when I didn't want to be a doctor. The decision came easily and early, the journey to get there long and arduous. At the age of six I was free-handing a drawing of the heart. At ten I was observing people with rashes, different gaits, bandages, and abnormal features, wondering what it was they had and how I could make them better. This is not meant to sound self-serving; it's simply who I was at the time. I was fascinated with illnesses, what caused them, and how to treat them. At fifteen I was working with a Philippine surgical team in Laos, actually present in the operating room and assisting in surgery (and I don't mean just holding retractors), learning to suture, and observing human anatomy firsthand. I did this during every break from school: fall, Christmas, spring, and summer. This informal but hands-on kind of education continued, so that I found myself in situations that offered opportunities not given to most, and I eagerly took advantage of them because of my father's position.

My time in Somalia holds many memories for me, most of which involved learning to be independent and feeling comfortable in a different culture. That would serve me well as I moved from country to country over the years, making it possible to fit in more easily with local customs.

Mogadishu wasn't very developed in 1958. There was a paved road that served as the main conduit for vehicular traffic, which was sparse, and dirt roads everywhere else. It was a small city with varying degrees of structured homes, as well as a lot of village huts. We lived in a simple house provided by the U.S. government, had a Land Rover, and went to school by way of correspondence courses in somebody's house where one of the diplomat's wives—a teacher—lived. Elementary students studied in the living room, middle school kids in the kitchen, and one or two high school students were left on their own. There were twenty children max. We'd all be picked up by a school bus in the morning—nothing more than an American Embassy van—and would learn from 8 a.m. until noon. After midday, it got so hot that we weren't able to be very productive when it came to studying. Even the American Embassy and USAID closed down because of the heat. So I went back home, ate lunch, and took a little siesta in one of our bedrooms, which had the only air conditioners in the house. Around three or four in the afternoon, we always set off for the bush—a short fifteen-minute drive outside of the city—to hunt or see the wild animals. This was my routine until I was twelve years old. It was radically different from growing up in the suburbs of an American city and afforded me a cosmopolitan view of life.

From Somalia we moved to Tunisia, and at twelve years of age I was in the 8th grade. I attended the American School for all embassy and USAID families. There were eight of us in the 8th grade class: four boys and four girls. When we graduated, seven of us went to boarding schools in Europe, and one went to a boarding school in the United States. My father was transferred to Laos in 1964, where he was stationed for the next twenty years. It was in Laos that I really began my journey into medicine.

Vientiane, the capital of Laos, was a busy little city, with a culture quite different than what I was used to in Africa. The people were more open and more engaging. They were quick to speak and to share their lives and opinions. It was an easygoing culture. Laughing and smiling were the norm, which represented a departure from the stoic, hardened character of the Somali. For the Laotian, everything was laissez faire: no worries, no problems, no anger. Car accidents yielded laughing drivers as they recounted how the accident happened, making fun of each other in an non-accusatory way, blaming no one. And off they would go, melting back into the mainstream of Laotian life.

In the northern part of Laos, however, where the culture espoused a more serious mindset, things were different. The Hmong (also known as the Meo) and Akha tribes were isolated, fiercely singular and protective of their land and property. Luang Prabang, the royal capital, was rich in history, with a cultural tapestry that was unique to the city. Embraced by mountains on all sides, Luang Prabang was majestic in its own right, a showcase of untouched beauty protected by the forbidding terrain. I grew to love that city. We traveled there a few times every year to attend royal functions, my father representing the U.S. government. I met the king of Laos, danced the lamvong, a traditional Laotian dance, with the king's daughter—she was my age—and rode in royal processions as a distinguished guest. The first time I experienced this, I was fourteen. I found myself drawn to the beauty of the people and the country. I learned their culture and observed the characteristics and mannerisms of the Meo and the Laotians. It prepared me for later years, when I returned to Southeast Asia as a physician, this time in Cambodia. Or perhaps I was there because God was preparing me for what He had in mind for my life. I now firmly believe that He was tapping me on the shoulder to get my attention.

I also had an affinity for flying. I still looked up at the sky every time a plane flew overhead, just as I'd done when I was six. I somehow knew I was going to pilot a plane one day. At our home in Vientiane, there were two fans in the living room, each spaced about four feet apart on the ceiling. The controls for each were side by side on the wall facing the entrance to the living room. I could stand at the controls and face the fans, seeing them easily. I would pretend to start "engine number one" by turning on one fan before starting "engine number two" by turning on the other. The controls had numbers on them from one to five—slow to fast. Turning them, I'd make them go faster, accelerating down the runway for takeoff. I was thirteen years old, and it seems silly to speak about it now, but it set the tone for my desire to fly. Today, when I push the throttle of my plane forward for takeoff, I still see myself standing in that living room, turning those fan controls full right to number five. God was again preparing me for things to come—again tapping me on the shoulder.

Air America was an airline (if it can be called that) dedicated to the service of Southeast Asia and was later identified as a "CIA airline." I got to know it well. C47s would fly from Bangkok to Vientiane and back carrying supplies and passengers, mostly U.S. embassy and USAID personnel. I loved that airplane. It and the DC-3 are still my dream planes. I would often sit in the cockpit with the pilots, who got to know me, and I would ask question after question. When we flew from Vientiane to Luang Prabang and back, it was always with Air America, which had daily scheduled flights up and back called "milk runs." Without getting into too much detail, on rare occasions I'd be allowed to sit in the right seat and put my hands on the yoke, my feet on the rudder pedals. There would be a gentle turn to the left here, a cautious bank to the right there, with a steady hand by the captain in the left seat always helping, guiding, and teaching me. I learned to "feel" the airplane and let it become a part of me. There were no post-9/11 restrictions back then, only an open cockpit to all who were curious and interested, with pilots who were excited to have a young teenager worship them. Let's just say that when it was time for me to take formal flying instructions and get my pilot's license when I returned to the U.S. to go to college, my instructor and I flew around, going to breakfast and lunch just to build up hours in my log book to meet the minimum number of hours flown in order to get my license. I got my pilot's license at eighteen but had learned to fly at the age of fifteen with some of the best stick-and-rudder pilots there ever were. I still prefer to hand-fly my plane if conditions permit rather than using the autopilot since I can sense the plane as an extension of myself.

I'd be doing a lot of flying as an adult, and I would return many times to third world countries as a doctor. Everything up to this point in my life had served as a prologue to chapters in my life that were already being written, chapters that had been outlined while I was living abroad with my father. While I knew that I wanted to go into medicine, I didn't yet know how everything would eventually play out, although there was someone who did. I would return the States, and when I did, the Author was going to have a few things to talk about with a somewhat self-absorbed medical student—with His work in progress.

Chapter Two
Taps on the Shoulder

College, medical school, pediatric residency, and a pediatric critical care fellowship came next. A few people came into my life that made a big difference. Dr. Samuel Gray III, a cardiologist, showed me what it meant to be a compassionate physician. He taught me to listen to patients, to feel comfortable sitting at the bedside while holding a hand, and to always put "care" in focus while doing my best to "cure." He came into my life when I was a medical student, a time of idealism, unrealistic expectations on my part, and excitement about being a god in a white coat.

At that time, however, I was young and extremely aggressive in the management of my career. As a god in a white coat, I thought I knew more than everyone, believing I could cure anything. I certainly felt invincible and that I was making a difference in the lives of many people, and I wasn't hesitant to take credit for it. It was all about me, and I sought out the attention and the accolades that came with such godlike territory.

During my last year of residency, I joined the International Rescue Committee as medical director of the pediatric ward at Khao I Dang refugee camp on the border of Thailand and Laos. This was during the Khmer Rouge genocide that killed over 2,000,000 Cambodians. On December 23rd, 1979, I arrived at Khao I Dang, It was at the bottom of a mountain range, where Cambodia lay—and where millions of people murdered by Pol Pot's forces now rested. I walked into the camp silently, smelling the dust and the death. The hospital camp was being built, bamboo shacks lined up one after the other, each assigned to a different international medical team. There is something palpable about death, and I literally felt it before I actually saw it. I heard a gasp from a nurse who was in my team and followed her eyes to the top of the mountain range above us. The mountaintop was lined with thousands of refugees, standing, sitting, and lying down, all of them plaintively looking at us. More appeared, pushing those who were in front down the mountain. We heard gunfire, sporadically at first, and then constantly. The refugees didn't run or panic. They just kept gathering at the top of the mountain range. Some fell and didn't get up, while others turned and looked back towards their homeland. Those same refugees would never return there, and many would shortly die.

I slowly backed away from what I knew was about to happen. Within moments, the side of the mountain was filled with thousands of refugees running towards our camp, but we weren't prepared. In fact, we hadn't even unloaded our medical supplies yet. The only medical team that was close to being settled was the German trauma unit. Fortunately, they were skilled at handling such a scenario. Within minutes, the camp was filled with refugees, and in the first ten minutes I saw three people die. We struggled to set in motion an organized triage system, but this quickly failed. Within three hours, we had over 10,000 refugees in our camp. By the next day, we had 21,000 refugees. Within three weeks, we were up to 65,000, and after three months, we had 150,000 refugees. That first day, over 650 people died. By the second day another 600 had died, and by the end of the week we were seeing, on average, 100 people dying each day.

I had seventy to one hundred children in my ward, and I had to make painful decisions as to who would live and who would die. The Red Cross simply couldn't provide the necessary supplies and equipment given the sheer number of refugees. A woman whose husband had just died looked at me with pleading eyes, having traveled treacherous miles so that an American doctor could treat her dying child. I had no words to explain that I didn't have the necessary equipment. Because of the lack of supplies, only emergency surgeries were performed, and we had to fight to do routine appendectomies. Some cases remained untreated, such as a young child with pneumonia.

The human suffering was incalculable. Because of the steady influx of refugees, arrangements were made to move some to smaller camps, and many people awoke in the morning not knowing where they would be at the end of the day. This resulted in many families being torn apart since people were coming into the camp and leaving at a dizzying pace. Returning to their homeland and taking their chances with the Khmer Rouge wasn't much of an option, and by the same token, they risked being shot by neighboring countries who didn't want to be burdened by refugees. As for Vietnam, it was chaotic and not much of an option either.

At the end of my three months as medical director of the pediatrics ward at Khao I Dang, I was amazed at how much could be accomplished by making a diagnosis using only my eyes since sophisticated diagnostic equipment was limited or totally unavailable. It was also the first time that I lost respect for a culture due to the thousands of skeletons piled high in the region. I had grown up in an atmosphere of tolerance, but the shadow of death hung over Southeastern Asia for many years during and after the Vietnam War.

Cambodian camps leave their scars

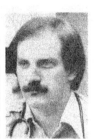

By LESLIE ELLIS
Courier-Journal Staff Writer

The first 10 minutes David Beyda was at the Cambodian refugee camp, he saw three children die. The disease, people dying by the hundreds and the inhumane living conditions eventually robbed him of his sensitivity and his empathy, and he knew it was time to come home.

When he left the camp, "things were on the verge of falling apart," Beyda said yesterday, as he sat in the physicians' lounge at Children's Hospital in Louisville and described the experience that has altered his ideas about medicine, himself and his acceptance of different cultures.

"It's going to get a lot worse before it gets any better," said Beyda, the son of

a former foreign service officer who works with the United Nations in Thailand.

Beyda, 28, returned to his job as a senior resident in pediatrics at Children's Hospital about a month ago. He had spent three months as director of a pediatrics unit at a refugee camp at Khao I Dang, where he said 120,000 people live in squalor that overpowers the senses.

Beyda is working with the International Rescue Committee to recruit physicians to go to the refugee camps so the medical care can continue.

At Khao I Dang he had anywhere from 70 to 100 sick children in his ward. Of those, at least 20 were critically ill.

"I found myself looking at four or five kids in the morning, and making a

decision on which one lives and which one dies," he said.

The children's families had been torn apart by the terroristic acts of political regimes in Cambodia.

He remembers how a Cambodian mother, her eyes pleading, told him that her husband had been murdered and that she had just traveled treacherous miles to get to a refugee camp in Thailand so her dying child could be treated by an American doctor. But there weren't enough medical supplies to treat her child. "How do you tell that to someone?" he said.

As a child, Beyda lived in Africa, Europe and Southeast Asia. He had a

See DOCTOR
Back page, col. 3, this section

When I left the refugee camp in June of 1980 I felt that I was meant to be not just a physician, but that proverbial god who is revered as he walks down the halls of a hospital. I was very self-serving and embraced the ego that I exuded so easily. When I walked into the foyer of Johns Hopkins, a high-powered academic institution, it cemented my god-like demeanor. I was there to complete my pediatric critical care fellowship, and it was a heady time. While I was at Johns Hopkins I became well known for my research in brain resuscitation. This precipitated the rise of my academic career, which included lecturing around the country. I became known for aggressive and innovative techniques for measuring the metabolism of brain cells, as well as blood flow to the brain. All of this further enhanced my image of a white-clad god, and my ego grew larger. At the end of my fellowship, I was heavily recruited to start a pediatric ICU. I chose Phoenix Children's Hospital, and in 1982 started their Intensive Care Unit. Over the course of several decades, my partners and I built it to what it is today: an internationally recognized pediatric critical care unit.

During those years, I continued to build upon my accomplishments and to lecture around the country. Then a series of events unfolded that would forever alter the trajectory of my career. I was forced to question my god-like status.

It started with a mother in the ER. She'd left Flagstaff late at night, her three-year-old buckled in his car seat in the back. Her husband reminded her to drive carefully, but the admonition wasn't heeded. Somewhere between Flagstaff and Phoenix she noticed in her rearview mirror that her son had managed to unbuckle himself and was trying to get out of his seat. She leaned back to secure him and lost control of her vehicle. He was ejected from the seat and sustained severe head injuries.

I cared for him as best as I could when he arrived at the hospital. There was nothing for me to do other than keep him comfortable, a frustrating task for any physician, especially one wearing a mantle of invincibility. His skull had been crushed and broken like an egg. When his mother arrived, she began screaming at me to do something. As compassionate and softly as I could, I told her that there was nothing for me to do. To a worried parent in the pediatric intensive care unit, such words are hollow. She began to strike me with her hands but abruptly stopped and looked at me, asking "Are you a Christian?"

"No," I said, perplexed at the non sequitur.

She slowly turned away and climbed into bed with her son and said, "God will decide whether he lives or dies."

I stood there, arms folded, angry at the question and her follow-up statement. Her sentiment wasn't part of my rational mindset. I myself was supposed to be the god she appealed to, a role I assumed without a second thought when I donned my white coat each day. I stayed angry, but a couple of phone calls several years later changed my approach to bedside medicine forever.

I received a call from the wife of Reverend Bob Stanley, pastor of the church that my wife and children attended. I attended, too, although I did it mostly as a token of family unity. The pastor's wife asked me if I would go to the hospital, where her one-week-old granddaughter had been admitted to the intensive care unit. When I arrived, Baby Nicole was already on life support, pale and weak. I cared for her over the next week while a rampant infection invaded her body, taking her organs one by one as if they were trophies. She was attached to monitors and a ventilator, tubes running into her small body and tubes running out. With each passing day, it became apparent that I wasn't going to win this one. I finally met with Reverend Stanley and the parents and told them that it was time to take Nicole off life support. The family understood, and I placed Nicole in her mother's arms and stopped the medications running through her veins. As I left the room, Reverend Stanley turned and said, "David, it's all about faith." I had no response and left. There was no way the baby was going to make it, faith or no faith. I'd tried to explore what faith meant on a few occasions, but hadn't gotten very far.

A few years later, Reverend Stanley informed me that he would be leading a men's retreat called "A Walk to Emmaus." Believing it might help me with my nebulous ideas on faith, he suggested that I register, although there was a two-year waiting list for this well-attended retreat. Surprisingly, I got a call shortly thereafter from a woman with the church saying that there had been a cancellation. Coincidence? Who knows? Einstein said that coincidences are God's way of remaining anonymous. Two weeks later, I came to Christ on October 26 1996 at four in the morning, and after that I was a different person. As time progressed I began to pray with my patients, trying to be humble and selfless according to the grace that He gave me. The god in the white coat was gone.

As for Baby Nicole, I would eventually attend her wedding after she'd graduated from college summa cum laude. Nicole—the baby I took off life support so that she could die—had no limitations or aftereffects from her time as a sick baby. As Bob Stanley tried to tell me, it's all about faith.

The first call that changed my life came in 1996. The phone rang again in 2004, and it, too, represented a milestone on my journey to a medical ministry around the world. I was unsure of the number, wondering who could be calling, but I answered it all the same. Don, a principal in the financial firm we were using, introduced himself and asked if we could have lunch to discuss the healthcare of children in Cambodia. He said he had been told of my past experience and wondered if I could be of help. Lunch it was.

It becomes evident from time to time that God wants us to feel the poke He gives us, and the lunch meeting was a mighty poke indeed. Don explained to me that he was on the board of a sponsorship organization called Mission of Mercy (MOM) and that they cared for several thousand children in Cambodia. He asked if I would I be interested in evaluating their health. He'd been meeting with a nurse named Kelly Ramsland, who had a heart for medical missions, and they were looking for a doctor to go to Cambodia. As I listened to Don, vivid memories of my time at Khao I Dang returned. Lettuce, cucumbers, and salad dressing mixing in my mouth as I chewed gave me a moment to think about what he was asking, or rather what God was asking. I was already many years into my role as Division Chief of Critical Care at Phoenix Children's Hospital and wondered how I could help. The time to do so would be elusive given my schedule, and yet the request touched old memories of my days in Somalia and Laos. This meeting with Don was on a Friday, leaving me the weekend to mull over his proposal.

On Saturday, the early morning alarm rang, and my wife and I both rose. It was customary for Charlcye and I to get up early, have coffee, and sit on our porch and spend some time reading or talking things over, waiting for the sun to command that our day begin. On this particular morning, we naturally had a lot to talk about. I brought her up to date on my conversation with Don and talked about how going to Cambodia would be a welcome change from what I was doing. It had been years since I'd gone to Sri Lanka to help build a cardiac ICU at Colombo General Hospital with my two colleagues, Dr. Jeremy, a pediatric cardiovascular surgeon, and Dr. Dudley, a pediatric cardiologist. We had started the Children's Heart Project (CHP), bringing pediatric cardiac care to a country that had a waiting list of over a thousand children who needed to get their hearts fixed. Regrettably, most died waiting. And there is one story that remains with to this day.

Idealism filled my mind and charity filled my heart as we travelled to Sri Lanka fulfilling a mission to teach, established a foundation upon which the local physicians could grow on and correct as many congenital heart defects as possible in the short time we were there. Aside from the primitive environment and the lack of sophisticated equipment other than what we brought with us, the types of heart defects we saw were no different from those we see here, the goals not unlike what we try to achieve in our country. What was different is that we cared for children who were malnourished, debilitated and headed for an early death. They were clutched and thrown into a river of medical expertise and technology that rocked them from side to side with each wave. Tension was thick; humor was the fashion and emotional outbursts predictable.

I remember one little girl in particular. She sat, legs crossed, hands clasped in her lap on a gurney, her mother at her side in pre-op holding. At ten years of age, she looked at me through eyes that have seen more than someone twice her age. She came to the hospital by bus, some two hundred miles away and months before our arrival to take her place in line. Her mother knew nothing about us, except that we could fix her daughter's heart. There is no question that this little girl had not been given a fair start at life. We were a hope, a second chance for life.

That very morning, I held her hand as she lived. Twelve hours later I would hold her hand as she died. Her mother thanked us for doing what we could, prostrating herself in front of us as if we were gods, behavior we seldom see in western medicine.

Deliberation about the risk of therapy is more than usually difficult, and this I think, is a concern worth taking seriously. The attitudes underlying the practice to do "good" for all our patients, seems not out of keeping with the spirit of healing that we all subscribe to. But nobody is at his best every day. And that includes those of us who call ourselves physicians. Despite our best intentions, we have on occasions, made either small or large errors in our practice. Although medicine is supposed to be a science, there is certainly a great deal of experimentation that takes place, which in itself is prone to error. To think that physicians are far from the common road traveled is to bask in the realm of idealism. This very human character which we possess is however, not readily accepted by our patients and their families, and yes, by our own colleagues at times. The feeling that lives are at stake lends credence that error is unacceptable. I attend particularly to how our patients are affected, not by neglect, but by day-to-day patterns of medical practice, decision making in particular: to risk therapy or not. But we do take risks frequently with our attempts at heroics. And despite some skepticism, we are more often than not successful. We celebrate life and watch the children grow, joyous in our triumph. But sometimes, we fail.

Challenges in medicine continue to center around technological, pharmacological and physiological advancement. We don't allow nor accept the status quo. And that holds true for battling mortality. The natural selection that Darwin proposed has never applied to the human population. Or at least medicine doesn't let it. Not to imply that we contributed directly to her mortality, but the thought often occurs to me that her life would have come to an end without surgery sometime in the near future. By operating on her, with her reserves depleted, we took a chance and perhaps cheated her out of some precious time that she would have enjoyed. A statement I make for discussion purposes only.

What about the fact that this little girl entered into a relationship voluntarily expecting to come out of surgery a little better than when she went in? What were her last thoughts before she fell asleep under anesthesia? Did she say a little prayer? Was she afraid or was she joyous that she was soon to have a new life? I can't begin to imagine what she thought. I just hope that it was pleasant and full of love. Her innocence could not allow her anything else.

I have an old think attitude when it comes to deliberating risks of therapy. And that is that virtue may be worth a good deal more than just the warm glow of satisfaction that comes with knowing you've done the right thing. As far as that little girl is concerned, I can find comfort that operating on her was the ethical thing to do, the human thing to do. We did the very best we could. That's all we knew how to do. But was the risk worth it?

We'd made over fifty trips during the ten years that we went, training local cardiologists, surgeons, and anesthesiologists to care for children with congenital heart abnormalities, and they built it up to include a separate children's hospital with a progressive cardiac program. Pediatric cardiac care improved, moved forward, and today there is a full-fledged pediatric cardiac program in Sri Lanka. Although CHP dissolved as an entity, we ensured the future of sustainable care before our work was finished.

There were sleepless nights that weekend since God was poking me again. By Sunday it was clear that I was going to Cambodia and assess the healthcare of the Mission of Mercy children. Kelly and I put together a small team, and off we went. Ten days later we came back and I reported to the president and the board of MOM that a more comprehensive and focused medical program would benefit their sponsored children. They, in turn, asked me if I would be willing to run it, and with Kelly we formed Medical Mercy. We would be responsible for the healthcare of 40,000 children in fifteen countries. The years ahead would be filled with trips on behalf of Mission of Mercy (now One Child Matters) as I and my teams helped the forgotten children whose faces had been erased by materialism and the frenetic pace of modern life. I don't think they would have come to pass, however, if I hadn't made the Walk to Emmaus retreat with Reverend Stanley.

While walking to the town of Emmaus shortly after the crucifixion, some of Jesus' disciples met a stranger on the road, and he began to talk about recent events in Jerusalem. When they later sat down to eat with the stranger, they recognized him as the resurrected Christ. He'd been there all along. I recognized Christ on October 26, 1996. I, too, can say that He'd been there all along.

Chapter Three

The Forgotten Children

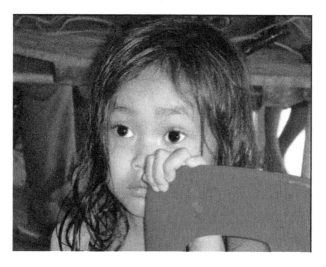

My life and priorities profoundly changed after Don asked me
to evaluate the health of children in Southeast Asia, and God's
purpose for me became clearer from that day on. I began a loose
association with MOM in November of 2004, taking a medical team to Cambodia, and I made additional trips in the years
that followed. I was convinced that I made the right decision to
bring my clinical skills to third world countries, which I came
to love so deeply when I was growing up. I resigned as Medical
Director and Division Chief of Pediatric Critical Care at Phoenix
Children's Hospital in order to follow God's command to serve
in countries where medical care was desperately lacking.

The schedule was hectic. With my Medical Mercy teams,

I made eight trips to Cambodia in a year and a half and made assessment trips to countries in need of medical care, such as Jordan, Gaza, Ethiopia, Egypt, and Swaziland. As a result, we began medical intervention programs in several of these countries. It was sobering to think that so many locations needed help in finding basic healthcare, but our teams took one step at a time in binding the physical and psychological wounds of those we'd been led to serve. In all, it had been a good beginning. We traveled with a Christ-driven purpose and moved in the direction He sent us, knowing that we were simply His servants. There was no place here for a god in a white coat, and thankfully I had abandoned that role long ago. Given the vast number of children we served, approaching our task with anything but humility would have been folly.

One Child Matters has a unique vision for a specific group of children who are largely forgotten by other child sponsorship organizations, and for this reason I call them "the forgotten children." This group is comprised of individuals who have slipped through the cracks, children not generally in the forefront of people's minds when they look at headlines and labels rather than the reality beneath the words. They are street children, children impacted by HIV/AIDS, victims of child trafficking, children of armed conflict, and those under five simply struggling to survive. In short, they're a ragtag bunch, pleading with pained expressions for recognition. Some have tears in their eyes; some remain silent. Many are depressed, suspicious, and oppressed by the conditions they live in. One Child Matters strives to remember these lost ones and to bring them forth from the shadows so that we can reinstate them into the human family

Every day, forgotten children are exposed to multiple

threats to their physical and mental well-being. They grow up without access to proper adult care and attention, and their lives are led outside of the protection normally extended to the young and vulnerable in most developed countries. As young and needy as they are, many are forced to look after themselves or assume the role of caretaker for their siblings. It's a crash course in survival, a course that many never complete.

The truth is that there are forgotten children and adults in *all* cultures. Think of an elderly patient in a nursing home whose relatives never visit. Or consider the patient in a psych ward who has no friends as he shuffles around the Day Room, his tenuous connection to reality being a game show blaring from a big screen TV on the wall. To be forgotten is tantamount to being excised from humanity. The plight of forgotten children is an extreme example of such marginalization because, in many cases, they have no parents, food, or shelter. Abused, used, and neglected, they are sometimes hours or days away from death. They don't have the amenities or security that the average child has in the West—no safety nets to keep their lives together. In the years ahead, I would encounter these children in almost every country I visited on behalf of One Child Matters. I would hold their hands, look into their eyes, say a prayer, and know that they are children of God, a Father who never forgets the least among us.

In March of 2006 I made an assessment trip to the South African country of Swaziland. It's slightly smaller than New Jersey and had a population at the time of slightly more than one million people. Four in every ten people in Swaziland were HIV positive, and the life expectancy was thirty-three years. Compounding this grim statistic, a third of all children were without parents. Half of the patients in the hospitals had AIDS, and an estimated 50,000 people died each year from the disease. Most AIDS victims never saw a hospital and died at home, usually alone.

I went to Swaziland to look at the medical treatment available for the forgotten children cared for by Children's Cup and Mission of Mercy. (Children's Cup is a humanitarian and spiritual aid organization that builds orphanages and provides food and medical care around the world.) There were 50,000 forgotten children there, and yet everyone in that large population had a face, a name, and a backstory. When I was growing up, Mahmoud taught me to observe situations closely, and I was now able to see the individual lives beyond the statistics.

As expected, medical care in Swaziland was far from adequate. The hospitals were antiquated, the equipment didn't work, and the facilities were dirty, crowded, and poorly staffed. Nursing staff was obtained from local training programs, which themselves didn't have enough teachers to educate the students, creating a classic Catch-22. There was no medical school in the country, and those who wished to become doctors traveled beyond the borders to receive medical training. Most never returned. The doctors who practiced in Swaziland were from Cuba, Zambia, Egypt, Ethiopia, and other countries. I wasn't able to determine the quality of their education nor their clinical competency, although I met an Ethiopian pediatrician who had a personal bias towards palliative care for children with HIV, citing the futility of trying to treat patients with HIV/AIDS, only to have them die anyway. That kind of attitude did nothing to foster encouragement considering the staggering need for qualified physicians in a land ravaged by HIV.

The first facility our team visited, Raleigh Fitkin Hospital, was a Nazarene-associated hospital, and there was confusion as to who actually owned and ran it. The second was Mbabane Government Hospital. The wards and the outpatient clinic were below standards even for a comparable underdeveloped country (Ethiopia for example). Physician availability was marginal—almost nonexistent in some cases—and nursing care was virtually absent. The Matron of Nursing shared with us that the nurse-to-patient ratio during the day was one nurse to twenty-five to thirty patients, and at night it was one to forty-five. This essentially eliminated the possibility for any substantive care whatsoever for a patient to whom a given nurse was assigned. The wards were crowded, and babies were lined up side by side on a table, with their mothers standing at their feet and no place for them to sit. The babies we saw ranged from one month to one year old, all with IV fluids running and all clearly in critical condition. We saw eight babies one afternoon, and when we returned the next day, we learned that two of them had died during the night. I asked the pediatrician about aggressive care for the babies, as it was clear to me that several of the infants needed additional care and intervention. He remarked that their intervention was "heroic," but it strained credibility to believe that this was the case. With no equipment available to do what he described, such intervention was impossible.

The outpatient clinics were always full. There was a VCT clinic (Voluntary Counseling and Therapy) where patients went to be tested for HIV, counseled, and started, if necessary, on anti-retroviral drugs (ARV therapy). According to the counselors staffing the clinic, the follow-up on these patients was admittedly lacking. Many patients never returned and therefore the number of people with HIV/AIDS, as well as the mortality rate, couldn't be gauged with any degree of accuracy.

It was clear that Swaziland would present a difficult

challenge for a Medical Mercy team given the shortage of staff and working equipment, as well as the large number of patients infected with HIV/AIDS. With the establishment of Medical Mercy Centers, referred to as Care Points, I thought we could address the healthcare needs of these children early enough to prevent the long-term effects of chronic or terminal illnesses.

Ray, a friend and brother in Christ, took my ideas on how a medical clinic should flow and put them down on paper. Ray is a well-known architect and produced designs for a Medical Mercy building that included two exam rooms, a nursing triage station, a waiting room for twenty patients, a lab, a pharmacy, storage, and two toilets. We therefore planned for our medical team to visit Swaziland in October of 2006. Our assessment indicated that trying to help orphaned children in this region would be a daunting task—maybe even an impossible one. I knew I was being called to help the people in Swaziland and stepped out in faith. With the plans for the Medical Mercy building having received Ray's special touch, I knew that good things could happen. Today it is a fully fledged medical clinic staffed by missionary nurses and local healthcare workers.

Chapter Four
Thankful for What We Have

Not all forgotten children are abandoned or live on the streets. There are those who are forgotten because they don't have the one thing that always commands attention, always summons goods and services, always renders people visible. It's money. Regardless of the currency, money is a universally recognized way of conducting transactions. It buys what we need to live, from food to electricity to healthcare. Money talks, and those who have it generally have more power than those who don't, which is not to say that it's a corrupting influence one hundred percent of the time. But here's the rub: some people have little or no money, and they are the ones who are forced pay a heavy price for their lack. Yes, they pay a price all right, but the currency they put on the table is costlier than the numbers people write on the front of a check. There are those who have and those who have not. In one of my earlier trips to Cambodia, I stared into the faces of a family that "had not" and underwent one of the most harrowing experiences I've encountered in medicine.

It's common practice in Cambodia for three to five people to ride on a small motorbike to get around. Usually it is a family, the father driving, a small one or two year old on his lap as he holds the handlebars, a toddler right behind him, and the mother on the back riding side- saddle. On this particular early morning, Samnang fell off the bike and broke both of her forearms and wrists in three or four places. A missionary happened to be in a truck directly behind the accident and stopped. He picked up the child, put her and the family in his truck, and drove them to the local hospital. He dropped them off for medical care and left. That afternoon he returned to see how the little girl was doing, only to find the mother wailing in the street, clutching her one year old, the father catatonic. The missionary asked where the little girl was and was led to a cot in a filthy hospital ward. Hundreds of flies were attached to her bandages, feasting. There lay the little girl, with both her arms amputated at the elbows. He was speechless. When he could talk, he grabbed the physician and demanded to know what had happened. The answer was simple.

"No money!" the physician cried, his arms waving in front of him, the irony of one who had arms and the one who was now armless painfully evident. "No pay! Cannot fix! Cut better!"

There had been no surgery to place pins, screws, and plates to fix the fractures. No money equaled no medical care. It was decided that the best thing to do would be to amputate the forearms as the surgery was quick and the care needed afterwards was minimal. No consent, no discussion, no remorse.

The missionary was our host for the medical team and came to the clinic, ashen and shaking, tears flowing as he told me the story. He asked me if there was anything I could do, and it was evident I needed to see the little girl and her family.

Evil things happen. Evil seeps into windows, under doors, and through vents. But was I personally ready to battle the kind of evil described by the missionary? I reminded myself why I was in Cambodia. I left the clinic and made my way to the hospital. I needed to see for myself, to hear for myself, to understand for myself that which seemed so incomprehensible.

By the time I reached the hospital it was dark, the heat and humidity still lingered, and the smell of sickness was strong. A building that had been whitewashed years before was now covered with green and blue mold patterned like a mosaic with no beginning and no end. The hospital, as much as it could be called one, had little light, on-and-off electricity, and small streams of water and sewage running along paths that led to the wards. I asked to see the doctor who had taken care of Samnang, and someone went to get him. The physician was devoid of emotion—abrasive, cold, and defensive. He met me outside the hospital, refusing to let me in. His eyes were stern, his glare unceasing yet calm in the way of men who'd seen enough sorrow but were no longer moved by it, knowing that others were better suited to the task of giving comfort. It may not have been who he once was, but it's who he had become. Without waiting for me to explain who I was, he told me there was nothing I could do and to leave. I did just that, if only to gather my thoughts and put into perspective what happened and why. Truth and decency were becoming silent casualties in my virtuous world.

I went back the hospital several hours later, the night moving past the midnight hour. I would argue my way in if told I couldn't enter but found no resistance from anyone when I arrived. The front of the building was masked by swarms of people squatting, waiting their turn to be seen. Many were silent, but others moaned in their pain and suffering even at this late hour. The dirt where they squatted was littered with garbage, leftover food, and excrement. Babies and young children lay on the ground next to their families. The filth and the smell gave birth to a wave of nausea, a kind I had never experienced before even in the most sickening places I had visited around the world.

I walked through the masses and entered the hospital, unsure of where to turn. Left, right, or straight—it made no difference. The entryway was filled with the sick, each lying on a bare cot with no sheets or pillows and surrounded by family members who kept vigil on the belongings of their loved ones. When it came to medical care for the ill, a prescription would be written for them, and it was up to the family to find the medicine, IV solutions, tubing, catheters—whatever was needed—and then buy them and bring them back for the nurse to administer. If the family had no money, the patient received nothing, waiting for the inevitable. I moved forward, scanning the room, not sure what I was looking for. Then, in the far corner of the room, I saw her: a little girl staring at her arms, a look of bewilderment on her face as she turned her stumps over and tried to grasp a spoon to feed herself. Her mother sat by her side, her eyes red from crying. I sat down beside the little girl and fed her, the mother resting her head on my knee. Neither had any emotion—no tears, no fear, and no anger. They both seemed devoid of person, of soul.

An hour passed, and I told the little girl that I would be back to see her. I was to leave Cambodia in a few days, and I told myself that I wouldn't let this event pass without making something good out of it. I retreated to my hotel room, cross-examining myself in the soft shadows of a moon coming through a single window as to what had happened and what might still be possible. An inner voice told me not to dwell on what I couldn't understand. I wasn't good at this. I was better at accepting the harsh reality of death, loss, and the consequences of having my patients linger due to heroic measures that shouldn't be taken. At such times I would lower my head and push on without looking back or wondering whether a second chance lay beneath the wreckage. But this was different. I decided to go back and tell them to do the best they could and live with the outcome. They didn't have the luxury of doing anything else. I wouldn't make false promises that everything would be all right because I knew too well that some things can't be fixed. No one could give Samnang her arms back.

I returned early the next morning. Her mother was again weeping silently, lying near her daughter's cot. I stopped and touched her shoulder, if only to let her know that I was there. She didn't move. She had a look of both hope and despair on her face. I moved to the cot. Samnang's eyes followed me, tears welling up, her lips dry and quivering. I looked into them and found something gentle and even forgiving there. It was innocence, and for the moment that was enough. I found it hard to be angry because I believe that what man has meant for evil, God will use for good. I had to believe that this little girl would someday find good in what had been done to her, for Samnang meant "good fortune."

I went to the bedside and sat down, Samnang's mother moving closer. There was a long silence while my mind ran through all the things I could say to them, things I wished could make a difference, but there was just too much that had happened that I couldn't explain. Samnang's case was about helplessness, submission, and abuse, so I did the only thing left to do: I prayed, silently at first, and then speaking softly, my hands on Samnang's head. Louder and more openly, my voice stronger, my heart was bursting. And then the tears came. All three of us—Samnang, her mother, and I—cried at what had happened. They were Buddhists, but they kept their eyes closed as I prayed. For a moment, I felt a great peace in knowing that one day Samnang and her mother might see this as a moment of grace and come to know Christ for who He is. I stayed there for a while and left as the moon overhead carried away the silence of a hurting child and mother.

I went back several times to see them while I was there with the medical team. The family grew stronger in their conviction to live with what they'd been given. Six months later, Samnang was fitted with a prosthesis for each arm, one I had arranged for her to receive even though it was rudimentary at best, with claws for hands.

I don't try to explain these kinds of events because they simply *can't* be explained. Some things in life just happen, and maybe they occur for a reason and maybe they don't. What I do know is that Samnang represented another category of forgotten children, forgotten because she lived in an impoverished country where healthcare was a commodity rather than a human good that all are entitled to.

In the Gospel, we are told that thousands of people with every kind of sickness imaginable were brought to Jesus. With few exceptions, they were the marginalized people of Palestine, outcasts who were not welcomed in the daily ebb and flow of society because they were considered unclean. They were forgotten, and like the have-nots of today, they were excised from the human family. But Jesus cured them all and never asked for payment from anyone. With God, no one is ever forgotten, and we are told that all are welcomed at His banquet table, not just the privileged few who "have."

One group that was especially frowned upon was lepers, who were forced to live outside towns and villages. In one instance, ten lepers approached Jesus, who sent them to the high priest. On the way, all ten found that they had been healed of leprosy. As nine of them proceeded to the priest, one returned to Jesus and threw himself on the ground, filled with thanksgiving and praise for God. He was thankful for being cured, for not being forgotten.

I won't forget Samnang, but that's my calling as I visit third world countries: not to forget.

Chapter Five

Even at Home

In July of 2006 I was making preparations for the team's trip to Swaziland in October. Teresa and Daran were there, and I was optimistic as to what we could accomplish. Teresa was one of several missionaries with Children's Cup, which cares for the forgotten children at the Care Points. Daran was overseeing the building of the medical clinic in Mbabane. The slab had been poured and the block walls were going up. As I lined up staff and equipment and prayed for the success of the trip, I thought of those people who suffer at home, people who were as forgotten as Samnang or the orphans we would shortly be serving in Africa.

I'd known Hugh for ten years. We met on the beach after I watched him for a few days as he talked to someone out in the ocean, always waving his hands and bowing. He spent days alone lying on a dirty blanket, always in the same place at the edge of the sand where it met the high tide. No one ever sat next to him, even when the beach was crowded. He wore the same clothes day in and day out, drank from a bottle in a paper bag, and had long matted hair and dirty fingernails. I found out later that the bottle was simply filled with water. I was intrigued by his actions, but embarrassed by the mindset of myself and others, which was avoidance and distrust. Hugh was a person, a "who," not a beach bum or a "what."

In the early evening, he would stand at the edge of the water, look west, bow, and lift his hat to nobody—at least no one that I myself could see. He would raise his hands, wave, and make the shape of a heart in the air, and I could hear him say "I love you" over and over again. He would do this until the sun sank behind the horizon, and then, with head hung low, he'd shuffle up the beach and disappear for the night.

I went up to him late one afternoon, introduced myself, and asked if he would like some company. Without any hesitation he said yes, and we met and talked for hours almost every day at the beach each summer. Hugh was sixty-four, had two Masters degrees, had taught poetry in college, and had lived *la vida loca*, high on LSD from the time he was twenty until he crashed at the age of forty. He'd been homeless on and off— more on than off. His mind was burned from the LSD, and his flashbacks were frequent, but during his lucid times he was smart, gentle, and humble. Sadly, these times were becoming fewer and fewer, and it was obvious that he was getting worse. He couldn't remember where he'd taught, gone to college, or when we saw each other last. He slept in a park off the beach.

I took him to one of our favorite places, Prince of Peace Abbey. We attended mass, prayed, and talked for several hours, looking at the ocean from atop a hill where the abbey is located. I listened as he moved from one subject to the next, sometimes making sense, most of the time not. We talked about Jo, who he saw and talked to on the ocean in the evening—his love, his life. He said she lived on a sailboat docked in the marina near the beach. I checked, and she didn't exist. I told him so, only to see his eyes water up as he became quiet. And yet he went on talking about her as if he hadn't heard me.

When I dropped him off at the park one day, I hugged

him, held his hands as we prayed, and felt comfortable being with him despite what he was: a homeless, wasted, lonely man. I'd grown to love him for who he was, a brother who sought only that to which he was entitled: dignity and personhood.

We look to others for love and support, welcoming the warm embrace of those we love and the softness of a touch—the smell, the feel, the words, and the look they give us with their eyes. Hugh looked to Jo for all of that as well because he believed in her. It was a fool's errand, but Hugh was a sweet, gentle fool who lived life as a consequence of what he'd done to himself. I looked past that and saw in him the forgotten children to whom we are committed—the innocent, abandoned, lonely, and forgotten children. Some are as close as a beach or the space beneath a bridge or overpass, and if they don't conform to our definition of normal, it's not a problem. We can label them as crazy and move on, ignoring their life stories. I think of Hugh often and hope that one day he'll find Jo.

And then there was Steven, who was seventeen when he died from leukemia. He struggled with life for several weeks while in the intensive care unit, and he and I had a fairly good relationship, sharing stories and simple hellos. His mother, however, was someone I couldn't relate to. She was angry, obstructive, abusive, and confrontational—and a Christian. She had incredible faith but little tolerance for reality. As a Christian I tried on many occasions to see past her faults and the abrasive way she treated us. I wanted to put my arms around her, pray with her, share scripture with her, and pray with Steven, but she wouldn't allow me to do any of those things. Her character and her demeanor prevented it, or so I thought. My pride and ego prevented me from looking past *what* she was and really seeing *who* she was: a mother experiencing deep pain as her son died.

I'd been on many medical missions, and there were more to come. Steven's case was a reminder that we would always be faced with people and countries that hate us, that don't want us there. There are situations I must look past, with Christ in my heart to help me accept the slap while turning the other cheek. I could have done that with Steven's mother, but chose not to. Sometimes the only thing to be done is to accept people for who they are, followed by the most humble prayer of all: Thy will be done.

Chapter Six

Gaza: A Place of Hurt

Our Medical Mission trips require a great deal of planning. We not only have to line up a team and secure supplies, but we have to know exactly where we'll open a clinic so that when we arrive we can get right to work. Since we operate in remote countries, advanced scouting is mandatory. Not all regions, however, are easily accessible—or welcoming.

The previous year, I traveled to Gaza on an assessment trip the day after I was in Amman, Jordan, the day the hotels were bombed. I was just a few hundred yards away from the bombs, visiting with an American missionary and pediatrician working in the refugee camps in Jordan. Gaza was an open sore, a wound that festered, an entire region that needed medicine that only true peacemakers can administer. It is a tangle of political factions, walls, barbed wire fences, checkpoints, and animosity. In one sense, I was looking to heal the hurt within the larger hurt. It is difficult enough to administer medical care in a country where poverty, disease, apathy, and economic depression are the driving factors behind illness. In a region like Gaza, longstanding political rivalries make serving those who need assistance that much harder.

Getting into Gaza was difficult. I traveled via the road to the Dead Sea, passing the baptismal site of John the Baptist.

I arrived at the border crossing only to find 1,000 cars lined up to get into Jerusalem. I used the pull afforded by American passports to advance to the front of the line, but realized that even with this advantage I would still have a long wait. I decided to use a VIP service that, for $82 per person, would fill out all the necessary paperwork and move me through this no man's land and into Jerusalem. It seemed like a good idea, so I paid a Jordan "departure tax" to leave the country. "No man's land" is exactly that: a five-kilometer stretch that belongs to nobody and yet is protected by everybody. I passed through no less than four checkpoints as well as multiple bunkers and armed sites. My passport were scrutinized at each checkpoint until I reached King Hussein Bridge and crossed the Jordan River into no man's land.

I arrived on the Jerusalem side at the Allenby Bridge checkpoint. Israeli security was very tight, a lot of questions were asked, and getting from Jordan to Jerusalem took me almost eight hours. There was a bomb scare on the Israeli side, and for a while I was told to stay put. Tension was everywhere, and the Israeli undercover agents were not so undercover. In plain clothes, they all carried Uzis and looked like they would not be hesitant to use them.

I finally arrived in Jerusalem and went to the Jerusalem Hotel for a late lunch, waiting for a missionary to take me into Gaza. He knew the ropes so to speak and would act as my guide.

When I reached the Gaza border, I found the city surrounded by huge walls, like Berlin was years ago. I got through three more checkpoints and passport controls before entering a bunkered tunnel. It was half a mile long, and I had to walk though, carrying all of my stuff by hand. The walls were riddled with bullet holes, and cameras were everywhere. I felt like I was entering a jail, and in a real sense I was. Gaza is indeed a prison since no one can go in unless they are with the UN or a non-governmental organization (NGO). I'd sent my passport information to the missionary weeks earlier so that he could get me clearance to enter Gaza.

No one could get out. Before the disengagement, 100,000 Palestinians from Gaza would go to work in Israel and return at night. Now they couldn't. Ninety-nine percent of all Palestinians were unemployed. Hamas ruled the streets, and the Palestinian Authority ruled the government—or what they regard as the government. Before the disengagement, there were approximately 6,000 Israelis living in Gaza on twenty percent of the land, with 1.4 million Palestinians living in the other eighty percent. Israel spent billions of dollars trying to protect those Israelis and finally disengaged from Gaza, pulling out their citizens. That land belonged to the Palestinian Authority. There are multiple refugee camps in Gaza that house Palestinians. Jabalia is one of them, and that is where we went.

I visited a school that taught grades first through third and had sixty students bused in daily from the refugee camps. It cost $40 a month to support a child, and they had full sponsorship from churches in the United States. Of the sixty students, only one was a Christian, although the three teachers were all Christians themselves. One Child Matters was attempting to start an after-school program for about 100 kids from the Zeitun area of Gaza. A former nursing school, it was very nice. The top two floors weren't being used, and I saw that they could easily be turned into a medical clinic.

I also noted that there was a lot of mental illness, depression, and bedwetting in children because of the atrocities they had witnessed. The refugees were so poor that many children were kept from school in order to sell peanuts on the street. Ironically, no one bought them because nobody had any money.

I finally reached the Jabalia refugee project, and it's difficult to describe what it was like. The buildings were simply shells, with as many as ten people living in small rooms without heat or electricity, although they did have water. I visited five families in all. Next, I went to a small dwelling where five severely mentally incapacitated women lived under the care of another elderly woman who had cancer. The poor and destitute seemed beyond hope. I met with two of the refugees, who themselves began an organization to get food and goods to the poorest of the poor. It was quite a testimony to their love of humanity.

In short, Gaza is a prison with walls. It is filled with people who have no hope, with children who are forgotten. It is a place of hurt. On July 8th, 2006, the Israeli army was only 500 yards from Zeitun, the refugee camp to which I wanted to take a medical team, but the war was heating up, and Zeitun was in danger of falling. The refugees that we met were in hiding, unsure of what was going to happen next. The forgotten children were hungry, alone, and scared. A team from Medical Mercy wanted to go, but couldn't. It was an example of a situation where nothing could be done. As was the case with Steven's mother, anger was the ultimate blockade, one far more formidable than stone walls and checkpoints, which were the symptoms and not the disease of political dysfunction.

There was real need in Gaza for a Medical Mercy clinic. The people there were suffering as badly as in any country I had visited, but the larger disease—the strife, darkness, and evil in the region—made establishing a clinic impossible. But couldn't God have made a way where there *was* no way, which he had done (and would continue to do for us) on so many occasions? Obviously he could have, but I had learned to walk in faith and not question when He closes a door. Faith is sometimes difficult to practice, for we inherently want to know why things are the way we are. There's always the urge to have things *our* way, especially when we see something that requires attention, such as the refugee situation in Gaza. I experience genuine heartache when I see an individual or an entire region that I am powerless to help. Seen from a different angle, however, life is easier when we let go of the reins and realize that His larger perspective can see the innumerable variables of a situation. In that sense, faith is liberating. We can step back and place whatever needs healing in His hands, knowing that the timing will be according to a better plan than any we can devise ourselves. This was a lesson I would have to relearn many times in the years ahead. My trip was therefore not wasted. I saw the needs of the children and refugees and gained valuable information, but I was reminded that I always have to follow His lead. It's always about faith.

As for Gaza, maybe another time—perhaps God's time. We'll be ready when the call comes.

Chapter Seven
Lifted Up on Eagles' Wings

In preparation for our trip to Swaziland, I spent the week at Makholweni Mercy Center in Swaziland, teaching a healthcare worker course I developed and watching the children who had been entrusted to our care. I examined a number of children and got a good idea of what we would be treating: malnutrition, abscesses, rashes, vitamin deficiency, and the consequences of HIV. Our medical clinic would be ready, a medical safe haven for the forgotten children and, as it says in the Gospel, a light on the lamp stand for all to see.

Over a five-day period of the healthcare workers training course, our workers learned basic anatomy, how to spot common illnesses, and administer first aid and CPR. By the last day they were able to do a full physical examination using a thermometer, blood pressure cuff, stethoscope, and pen light to examine the eyes, mouth, and throat. In five short days, these fifteen lay teachers became healers, God's instruments for the forgotten.

I was blessed by their love, commitment, and dedication. On the last day, they had me sit on a chair and then lifted me above their heads as they prayed. I was overwhelmed, broken, and humbled. I was lifted up. I'd come to teach others how to be His hands, His servants. At that moment, I realized to whom I really belonged. As the Michael Joncas song proclaims, "He will lift you up on eagles' wings."

We departed for our first clinic at Madonsa, Swaziland on October 10, 2006. Madonsa is a community on the northeast edge of Manzini. It's a very rural place, but because of its proximity to Manzini, it is becoming more urbanized. The community itself still has a rural Swazi feel, with most homes made of traditional stick and mud construction. By mid-afternoon we encountered our first medical emergency.

Pepe was a nine-year-old girl who was HIV-positive. She'd been diagnosed three years earlier and was on antiviral medication. Her mother had died of AIDS, and her father was close to death when we saw her. Over the course of several weeks, she'd been feeling ill, and she presented to the clinic with a temperature of 104, rapid respirations, and evidence of total body infection and pneumonia. Herpetic lesions in her mouth made it difficult for her to eat or drink, and she was therefore weak and dehydrated. We started an IV and gave her fluids and antibiotics. After bringing her temperature down over a period of three hours, she looked much better. We saw her again the next day and gave her the rest of her IV antibiotics. Pepe was close to our hearts the moment we saw her because she was an immediate reminder of why we were there. It says in Matthew Chapter 25 that whatever we do to the least among us, we do to Him. We had just begun, but already we saw His face in Pepe and the others that we treated. He was standing in our midst.

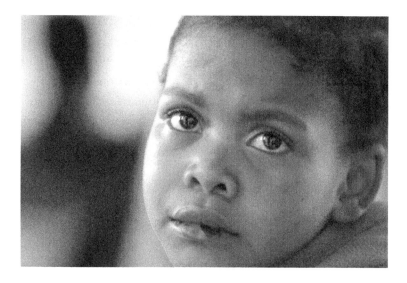

Medical Mission teams can assume many different faces, but they all have basic attributes in common, as was the case in Swaziland. Our typical team includes a medical team, sometimes a dental team, and an optical team to fit patients for reading glasses. Because there is so much demand for the services we provide, it's necessary to impose a certain amount of organization to maximize our efforts. Patients line up outside the clinic early in the morning and then register, with their names and addresses listed on an encounter card. After that, they proceed to a triage waiting line, where a brief medical history and vital signs are recorded. Patients are then moved to the appropriate waiting line for the service they are presenting for.

Medical Mercy believes that spiritual counseling is a number one priority since every trip we make is faith-based in an effort to serve those to whom He directs us. We require a local church (or church group) to commit to a follow-up plan before we agree to open a clinic. Ideally, the pastors of participating churches, together with their most mature church leaders, are present and actively pray with and provide spiritual counseling for patients. Our care is holistic and treats body, mind, and spirit. One thing we do not do is restrict medical care or medications if the patient is unwilling to participate in spiritual guidance and discussion. It is not for us to evangelize, coerce or force others to hear about Christ. We accept that God does what God does.

A pharmacist and pharmacy assistants distribute medications, and we also use a support staff from local churches and U.S.-based volunteers. There are always more people who want to help than we can accommodate, and we therefore assign roles to team members, working in shifts when necessary.

The day was rainy, and we arrived at Mangwaneni cold and wet. This was a community on the outskirts of Manzini, off the road to Mozambique, and was across the street from the city garbage dump. A high percentage of the community was unemployed, forcing them to scavenge for food and clothing in the dump. We saw Pepe again, and she looked better. Another round of IV antibiotics and IV hydration perked her up a bit.

The children seemed sicker and less happy. Simply put, there was a sense of evil in the area, a malicious spirit that was palpable to the discerning soul. We deal with issues of infection on every trip, but is it possible for an area to be spiritually infected with darkness, despair, and negativity? I believe it is, for evil is opportunistic and seeks to gain a foothold wherever it can, and misery and pain give it fertile ground to breed. Hope and faith were needed there more than anything else to bring freedom to the captive, for His power is greater than the power that lives in the world.

At the Ngwane Park Care Point the following day, the

weather started out cold and overcast, but by noon the weather was sunny, with not a cloud in the sky. The sense of oppression had lifted. There were a lot of medical issues to handle, but it was a time to thank Him for our blessings. We saw how tiny we were in the great scheme of things as we held the hand of a one-month old infant with pus in her eyes, comforted an old man trying to catch his breath between coughing fits, and looked into the eyes of a young woman who was HIV positive. She told us she would be dead in a year and asked if she could leave her three young children with us because there was no one to care for them. These were not the ordinary days we would have been leading back in suburban USA, where soccer practice, shopping malls, and sitcoms are the order of the day, but we knew we were in the right place.

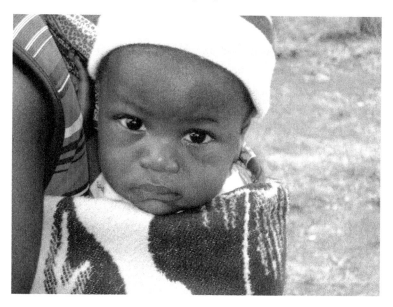

After Ngwane it was on to the new clinic in Makholweni, a word that means "the place of the Christians" because of the numerous churches located around the area. Despite this fact, most children there were left to fend for themselves. When we arrived, a thirty-eight-year-old woman presented with complaints of stomachaches. Two weeks earlier she'd ingested crushed bottle glass while trying to commit suicide. She'd learned that she was HIV positive and was ready to die. I sent her to see a spiritual counselor and heard that she came to Christ. Treating a deeper wound, such as the wish to die, is often the first step in treating the wounds of the physical body, and it is the reason we regard it as essential to work in tandem with missionaries and spiritual counselors. When we help bring someone to God, we perform the ultimate act of healing, although we never forget that we are mere instruments for the Spirit to work.

A woman approached me at Makholweni, her left arm dangling and her left leg dragging in the dirt. She stopped and looked at me, a smile slowly spreading across her face, the left side of which drooped from the stroke she'd suffered at birth. She waited not too far away, but not too close either. I smiled back and she came closer, her smile now wide and unrestricted, her eyes dancing. And then she collapsed. She fell to the ground, hitting the right side of her head, such falls having happened ten to fifteen times a day for years, her seizures barely controlled despite being on two medications. Teresa and I knelt beside her, protecting her head the best we could, trying to make sense of who she was and what was happening. She awakened after a few minutes, sat up, and leaned against the wall of the building. That's when I saw the lumps, bruises, and the swollen eye she'd sustained from her many falls.

Her story was one of many that drained me of my

expectations for humanity. She'd been this way since birth, cared for on and off by a mother, but mostly she was left to fend for herself. Four years earlier, a man in her village offered to help adjust her medications, feigning to know how to treat seizures. He lured her into his house, where he raped her.

There was one man who violated her, but there is one bigger than he who gives unconditional love, no questions asked. He loves her unconditionally, and I saw it in her smile. His unconditional love became hers, and that in itself is healing at its deepest level. May we be able to love like Him always.

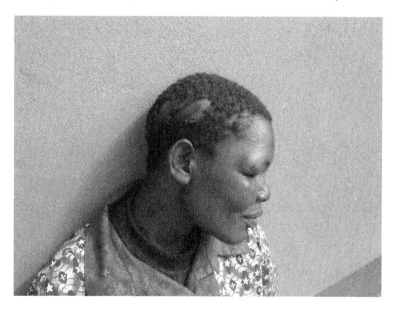

The trip was over, and the heartache lay in the fact that we couldn't do more in the limited time we had. We prayed that He would open the door for us to continue our missions in Swaziland. It is difficult work, but it is transformative for all involved, and that, I suppose, is the meaning of the New

Testament verse that many find elusive: anyone who finds his life will lose it, but anyone who loses his life will find it. The Medical Mercy team and I have found so much in Swaziland and the other countries we visit. We are indeed lifted up on eagles' wings.

Chapter Eight

Garbage City

There are times when we look in the mirror and ask ourselves why we do what we do. Most of the time the answer is ego-centered in nature: "Because I want to." We made a trip to Swaziland not because we wanted to, but because God asked us to go. We didn't question why, we didn't ask how, and we never said no. We just did it. We overcame hurdles and engaged in spiritual warfare in those places we suspected of harboring evil. We brought in the "big guns," and He led the way. It wasn't even a contest. We won. But St. Paul urged us to run the good race, and we would be heading to Cairo next, never satisfied to look over our shoulders and say, "That's done. Back to business as usual." My relationship with God meant that His business *was* my business for as long as He wanted me to serve the children of the third world.

Surrounded by fifteen-foot walls and isolated from the rest of the world, 200,000 families, making up a population of one million people, lived in garbage. In Cairo, Ezbet El Nakhel is aptly named Garbage City. The smell is powerful, the sights dramatic. Flies are everywhere, animals eat garbage, and donkeys pull carts loaded with even more garbage. It's everywhere. Children play in garbage, houses are filled with it, and raw sewage runs through the streets. In the midst of all this filth was another safe haven school for children. I went to Cairo to buy medicine and medical equipment and also meet with those who were overseeing the construction of our clinic on the fourth floor of the school. I wondered if it would be ready for our arrival since there are always logistical and organizational matters to attend to—meetings, discussions, emails, wringing of hands, prayer, and second thoughts—but unlike Gaza, the door seemed to be open despite the headaches that are part of our prep work.

Christ visited the house of Martha and Mary in order to teach. Martha complained that her sister Mary, sitting at the foot of Jesus and listening to His words, wasn't helping with the chores. Jesus' response? "Martha, Martha, you worry and fret about so many things, and yet few are needed, indeed only one" (Luke 10:41/JB).

Listening.

We listened to His voice and got ready to be His voice, heart, head, and hands in the midst of Garbage City.

He cleared the path, and we made it despite the obstacles in the planning stage. Every one of us had patients who touched us in a special way. I met a thirty-year-old woman who asked for help in having a male child. She'd been married at the age of fourteen and had two girls, one fourteen and another who was four. She'd had six miscarriages, all during the fifth and sixth months of her pregnancies. Three of those were males. When I asked her why she kept trying to have a baby after so many miscarriages, she said her husband wanted a son and that she was afraid to say no. I didn't have to ask her why she was afraid. I saw it in her eyes and in the bruises she had on her body. I had no way to help her since our missions don't offer fertility treatments. I asked her if she could leave her husband, and she looked down and simply shook her head. She was a Coptic Christian and a member of a very low societal and cultural hierarchy that has little respect for women. Prayer—silent prayer—is all that was allowed in her environment. She wouldn't pray with me and almost got up to leave when I offered to do so.

I wonder why people treat others the way they do, but I cannot judge, or so I am told. But I can sure ask questions, and maybe that's all that's needed for people to start judging *themselves*. I hoped that the woman would take a hard look at what she was allowing to happen in her life. I prayed that she would find solace in the love of Christ's grace that I told her was hers, no questions asked.

Lisa, a wonderful nurse on our team, had a special pregnant patient who wanted an abortion. She changed her mind after talking with Lisa, and such is the power of a faith-based ministry that looks at the entire person. Many doctors might have granted the woman's wish without a second thought, regarding it as a medical procedure and nothing else. Lisa was able to look at a much bigger picture, and because she did, a child of God would be born, open his eyes, and see the sunrise one day. And who knows? One day the child might be destined for great things. If not, simply growing up, falling in love, and having a family will be a miracle born from a brief talk with Lisa. Besides, being allowed to see the sun float above the horizon is pretty great in itself.

God spoke, and the pregnant woman, figuratively at the feet of Jesus, had listened.

A woman with breast cancer told Dr. Troy, a dedicated Christ driven physician, that she was ready to die because Christ was waiting for her. While it is always difficult to lose any of our patients, we're grateful that she had Dr. Troy to speak with, sharing her hope to be reunited with the author of all life. And who is to say that such an end to her story does not also represent a healing? God touches those we meet with much more than medicine.

In Garbage City, I looked into the eyes of two men who had aged gracefully and were still full of life, both without complaints and thankful for who they were and for what they had.

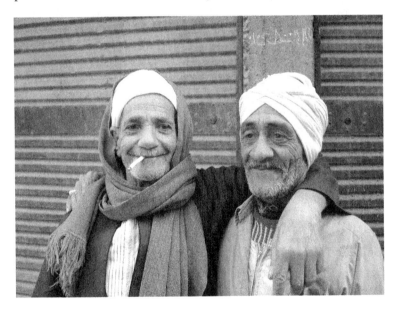

Their entire lives in Ezbet consisted of collecting garbage, sorting it, living in it, eating it, and sleeping in it. They made a living of fifty cents a day—if that—eating what they could find and living in a shelter made of old burlap bags and cardboard boxes. They had been friends for over fifty years and had no family other than each other. They were partners, pals, brothers, and soul mates. I spent several hours with them simply because I wanted to and, more importantly, because they made me smile. Despite their hardships, they had an outlook on life that is wanting in most of us: they were happy with what they had. Never once did either one of them complain about his situation. Rather, they shared their excitement in having another day to live with those who they loved—and with God on their side.

I confess that I challenged them for what seemed to be a cavalier attitude. I was, after all, on a mission to help people improve their lot in life. How could they live like this? Indeed, *why* would they live like this? Why didn't they go to the city and find a real job, get a real house, and live a normal life? They, in turn, challenged *me*. "What do you do with all your money?" they asked. "Where is your family and why aren't they here with you? Why aren't you smiling all the time? Why do you need to come here to see us in order to see yourself?"

So why *did* I need to go all the way to a Cairo slum in order to see myself more clearly—me, the man taught to observe people so closely by Mahmoud years earlier? Maybe it's because without the experience of seeing people like them, I see only what I want to see and avoid all that is unpleasant, blurry, and faded. At Phoenix Children's Hospital pediatric intensive care unit, we see awful things, but many times we look away or add another layer of paint to the picture in order to hide the sadness, such as a twelve year old—bald, weak, and pale—dying from cancer. It's all in how we view our lives, but once we look at ourselves as being blessed and gifted with various talents, no matter what they may be—even collecting garbage—we can begin to feel that we are, in point of fact, just that: blessed and gifted. Those two old men certainly felt that way, and I finally understood the meaning of their question. I had been tapped on the shoulder and told to listen, and through these men He spoke.

I was glad I'd met these two joyful men, who moved my spirit. It wouldn't be the last time that the healer would be touched by those he was sent to heal.

Muslims came to the clinic on the second day. Word of our presence had spread, and Nabil was asked if the clinic was just for Christians. He said it was open to all. They came and we witnessed to them as we would have for patients in any country. Not surprisingly, they "listened," for our prayer remains that He will send us those who have an open mind. A nineteen-year-old Muslim girl came from her sister's wedding that was taking place next door. She wanted to have fairer skin and to gain weight. We told her she was beautiful just the way she was. I believe we shared grace in affirming that she is loved the way she is.

Our last day in Garbage City was especially foul, with the smell almost overpowering, the dirt and dust causing many patients (and the team as well) to wheeze and cough. We saw an elderly man who had no breath sounds at all, ready to collapse. Thankfully we had a nebulizer and broke the attack with some albuterol. Several patients came to pray with us, and many more came simply to tell us their stories. This was especially touching, for it showed that our presence was recognized and that our reach extended far beyond the clinic. These visitors represented continued validation that we're always in the right place at the right time. And when a Muslim mother put her little daughter on my lap, I knew we were where we needed to be.

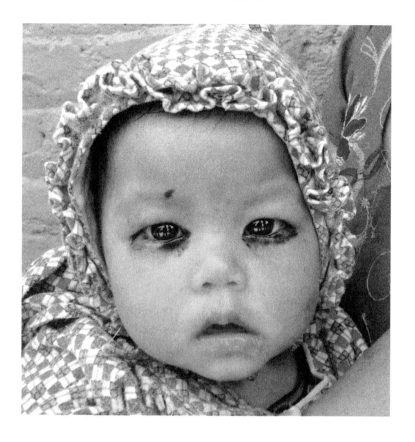

The medical clinic at the Joy School at Ezbet El Nakhel was a success, with Muslims and Christians together under the same roof for prayer, treatment, and fellowship. After we left, the clinic was staffed with an internist and a pediatrician every evening of the week from five to nine. There was ongoing medical and spiritual care for all who sought it. It was gratifying to know that our work would be continued long after we departed. We had planted seeds that He would continue to water . . .

. . . because we had listened.

Chapter Nine

A Jew, a Christian, and a Mennonite

After returning from Egypt, some of us left for Swaziland to work at Care Points and do an assessment for a possible medical clinic in Mozambique. I then made assessment trips to Honduras and the Dominican Republic in May of 2007. It was after the Swaziland-Mozambique medical mission trip in March that I paused one day to reflect on why things are the way they are in the world. I looked around and wondered why conditions weren't better. People died from AIDS in Swaziland, the residents of Garbage City lived in poverty and filth, the people of Cambodia were maimed and broken, and the children I took care of in the intensive care unit at home were sick and always trying to die, as I frequently put it.

There are many reasons why things happen, but more often than not, no explanation is forthcoming, as was the case with Samnang, and it was this fact that caused me to think about the suffering all around me. When I met AIDS patients in Swaziland, a sick girl with garbage on her feet in Cairo, and a man who'd lost his legs from a land mine in Cambodia, I thanked my lucky stars for what I had: a nice home, a good income, a wonderful family, and food on the table. But this was the "what" of David Beyda, not the "who."

On my trip to Honduras, I received more clarity on the "who versus what" of an individual. I saw a Hassidic Jew and his young son put their prayer shawls on and pray openly at the airport in Houston. Then I met a local pastor in Honduras who had a shofar (a ram's horn) that he blew every Friday in church before the Sabbath, and he blew it for me as he and I recited a classic Jewish prayer. On my way home, a family of Mennonites sat across from me at the airport in Honduras, praying from a book that I didn't recognize. In each case, I was seeing who these people really were. On the outside, the "what" was slightly different in each case, but at a deeper level everyone was somehow joined to God, to love, and to each other.

St. Paul says in Galatians 3:28 that "There is neither Jew nor Gentile, neither slave nor free, nor is there male and female, for you are all one in Christ Jesus" (NIV). Underneath our differences, we are connected as children of God, whatever we might call Him. That is our "who," our most fundamental essence. This truth began to shed light on the question of why there is so much suffering in the world, for when we choose to recognize suffering—when we stop looking away from it, as painful as that can be—we realize our interconnectedness. Everyone's suffering becomes our own suffering since the superficial distinctions we use to define ourselves fade away like so much smoke. And when we are brave enough to own the suffering of our brothers and sisters in Christ, we can carry out His command to heal, transform, and redeem. Acknowledging suffering cures our spiritual blindness and allows us to become who we are meant to be. I had wondered why I saw so much misery on my trips, and the diverse prayers I saw as I traveled to and from Honduras helped me to understand that St. Paul was looking past the "what" to tell us who we really are, or should I say *whose* we really are.

God receives prayers from many different faiths. I suspect He listens better than we do and responds in His own way. A Jew, Christian, and a Mennonite—how different and yet how similar.

Chapter Ten
Contrasts

I took a team back to Swaziland in June of 2007 to treat children at Care Points located at Ka Khosa and Logoba. According to locals, Ka Khosa is a community where prostitutes and thieves are made, a community where alcoholism, drug abuse, and child abuse are rampant. Prostitution, crime, poverty, and unemployment—an unsavory recipe that impacts children anywhere—all plagued Logoba, which had 15,000 people.

We visited two hospitals filled with abandoned children. All were physically disabled or mentally handicapped and lived in the laundry room. We saw a number of children who were very sick and cared for by their mothers, but we never saw a single nurse or doctor. Think about it: a hospital with no doctors, and a laundry room stuffed with handicapped children and their mothers like so many pieces of unwashed bed linen. It was as if the children were not only abandoned by their families, but by society itself. The atmosphere was surrealistic inasmuch as there was a healthcare setting with no staff to treat anyone—a horror story with a plotline worthy of a Stephen King novel. If there were ever any doctors or nurses there, even their ghosts didn't make themselves known. It was a strange contrast: there was a building designated as a hospital, complete with patients waiting to be seen, and yet no one was practicing medicine.

Imagine people in the United States arriving at an airport with no planes—no arrivals and departures—having only the expectation that a flight would occur because the building was called an airport. It would never happen. But such was the plight of the forgotten in Swaziland. They sat in "the hospital," hoping against hope that something—anything—might happen, hoping that maybe a doctor or a nurse might make a token appearance.

At Logaba, we examined 300 patients and saw interesting pathologies: subcutaneous larva migrans (crawling worms under the skin), weird rashes, heart diseases, and varying degrees of malnutrition. The wind picked up in the afternoon, and we were forced to see patients amid rolling clouds of dust. Children coughed and wheezed, and the nebulizer got a good workout. Just another clinic day in Africa, where the elements sometimes fight us as much as the diseases we're up against.

On the following day, we started out in the rain at a small Care Point in KaKhonsa called Gigi's Place. There were 300 patients, one tent, and a lot of dirt. The rain stopped and the wind began. Another contrast. The tent broke apart, the dust covered us again, and still the patients came despite the harsh elements. And why not? They lived in an area where the hospital was of no use, its laundry room a refuge for the disabled and downtrodden. Healthcare with no health . . . haves and have-nots . . . rain and dust—Swaziland was a place of extremes and paradoxes. Still, we did our best to treat AIDS, end-stage cancer, TB, malnutrition, and many other diseases—even a man whose leg was so badly infected that his sore was open to the bone. Thankfully, we saw Pepe again, who seemed to be doing well, and that made our hearts glow despite the weather and general environment of crime and neglect.

Crime, poverty, drugs, and prostitution. Despite these

sociological elements—diseases in their own right—we provided our own contrast by offering the forgotten a safe haven where they could be loved and cared for regardless of what was happening in the larger community.

We spent our last night at the Hlane game reserve. There was a full moon, native dancing, and the sound of roaring lions close by as we slept. The drive through the preserve brought us close to big game and showed us sites we may never see again. Africa is beautiful, wild, and yet filled with sadness. I can only wonder at the juxtaposition of such great beauty with need, disease, and death. The harsh law of survival of the fittest governs the wild, but it seems that this law operates among the human population as well: social Darwinism. Many advocate that we turn our backs on the incredible suffering in Africa and allow the have-nots to die out. If we ignore the suffering, the reasoning goes, nature will take care of hunger, abuse, drugs, and poverty without anyone lifting a finger. It will all disappear, and there will be no more contrasts, only lands of plenty where those once in pain have died out, having become as ghostly as the doctors that should have been in the hospital we visited. But this is not His way. All are invited to His table, including the poor, downtrodden, and lowly. Christ said that children were closest to His Kingdom and that it was His Father's will that not a single one be lost. For me, turning away is never an option.

On the way home, Glasgow Airport was shut down because of terrorist threats, and London was on high alert. It therefore took time getting through security. It was yet another odd and disturbing contrast: we were helping forgotten children while others tried to destroy human beings with senseless acts of violence. It made no sense, but then again, maybe we ourselves are responsible for the contrasts. If we turn away from the sick and dying, do we not create a self-fulfilling prophecy? Do we not ensure a widening gulf between the haves and have-nots? Or if we perpetuate war and violence in the name of cultural, ethnic, and religious differences—the "what" of who we are—don't we create a world of contrasts that speaks of "us against them"? Perhaps the deeper contrasts in life, the ones that divide or create strife and misery, are products of our egocentrism. We seem to have less appreciation these days for diversity. As for those who insist that progress is only achieved when people pull themselves up by their bootstraps, they forget that most individuals in underdeveloped countries don't have a boot.

Only He knows the ultimate reason why such contrasts exist, but I suspect they're prevalent in the world so as to make it easier to spot that which needs attention, that which begs for His mercy, grace, and healing. It is said that no man can serve two masters. Again, a contrast. Contrasts can restore our sight, but only if we dare to open our eyes and decide which master we will follow.

Chapter Eleven

Say It Ain't So

Our team went to the Dominican Republic at the end of August, 2007. With Hurricane Dean having recently skirted the island, everything was wet. There was a lot of rainfall, flooding, and power outages, but we nevertheless traveled fifty minutes from Santiago to a rural city called Moca and started our clinics at a Child Development Center named Niños de Dios, or Children of God—an apt name for the patients we'd be seeing. We couldn't go into the barrio or slums where the children actually came from since these areas, too, were full of drug trafficking, prostitutes, and crime. Given these conditions, it wasn't surprising that they harbored many forgotten children.

It was hot and crowded, but we marshaled on, seeing a little girl whose fingers had been sliced open and who had been taken to a local hospital, where her fingers were sewn up with old silk thread. When we saw the girl, her fingers were necrotic, or dying. We sent here to a better hospital, which fortunately was able to save her fingers. We also treated a boy with severe vitamin deficiency and what I thought was a variant of Marfan's Syndrome. The local people had given him the nickname Fish Boy. He got high fevers and needed to be put in tubs of water to cool off, and thus his name. Given cultural differences, the label probably wasn't intended to be derogatory, but the term Fish Boy nevertheless reflected the level of care in the region. The child had become a "what"—a Fish Boy—rather than a "who," someone with a name reflecting pride and dignity.

The hot, cramped conditions wore us down a little faster, but we didn't get discouraged. We were thankful that we could establish dignity in a dark area that needed God's light.

Pastor was a tall man of big stature, but he was gentle in heart and mind. I spent an hour with him, watching him struggle with debilitating pain. It had been two years since he'd first felt a tingling in his legs, followed by numbness, making it difficult for him to walk. He said that the pain was unbearable and that when he preached on Sundays, he leaned on God and the pulpit for strength. I watched as he struggled to get to his feet when I entered the room, and tears came from his eyes when he talked about the hardship of the last two years.

After the tingling and numbness had started, he'd seen several specialists, including an orthopedic surgeon and a neurologist. He also had a CT scan of his back, which was read as a herniated disc between L5 and S1. A nerve conduction test on his legs revealed little motor function or nerve input. He was told that nothing could be done and that he would soon be paralyzed from the waist down. He was given a prescription for Decadron (a steroid) and vitamin B6, which he was told to inject into each ankle every other day to help delay the paralysis. He did this for two years, spending all he had on tests, medicine, and syringes and leaving him no way to support his young wife and four-year-old son. Pastor was only forty-six, but he'd absorbed a level of pain that most people don't experience in a lifetime. He had just started a new church, and One Child

Matters had found a sponsor to build the school and support structures for over a hundred forgotten children. His ministry was moving forward, but he himself wasn't.

I examined him, confirmed that he indeed had severe neurologic injury to his legs, and that he was close to paralysis. I asked him to give me all of his medical records and that I would meet with him again after I reviewed everything. We prayed, and he was carried out to a waiting car. I then spent an hour going over his CT scan, nerve conduction tests, and reports from the orthopedic surgeon and the neurologist and found that the herniated disc was, in fact, treatable. I don't believe the pastor's doctors genuinely cared about him since he was a poor man and had little to offer in terms of payment.

As I was putting away his records, I came across a chest X-ray that had no accompanying report even though the film revealed an enlarged heart. No one had told him about this, and he wasn't being treated, although his wife told me that he'd suspected there was something wrong with his heart. He'd gotten an electrocardiogram a year earlier, but it had never been read. For a second time, a test on Pastor had been ignored, leaving him sick and in pain. I made arrangements for him to get additional studies so that he could receive care and surgery for his heart.

We arrived at Hosa, and I was told that Pastor was excited and happy that we were going to meet again. He knew I had news and that we could help him. His wife called a taxi, and as they waited for it they prayed, sang hymns, and talked about how the pain and suffering would soon stop and their ministry and love for the forgotten children would continue. As they prayed, the taxi arrived. His wife Daisy later told me that as they prayed, her husband called out her name. When she opened her eyes, his hands were curled, and he was blue as his large body collapsed. The waiting taxi took him to the hospital, where he was pronounced dead half an hour later. We received the news a few minutes later, and given how close Pastor had come to treatment, all I could utter was, "Say it ain't so."

I went to the hospital and spoke with Daisy, and she said that Pastor was the happiest she had seen him in years, knowing that we were hopeful he could be treated. He could hardly wait for the taxi to arrive. I struggled with whether or not I should tell Daisy what I'd found: that there was a good chance that surgery would have worked. He could have walked and been free of his pain, but no one had picked up on his heart condition. Would that make it worse for Daisy? I decided to tell her, and she listened, tears falling. We cried, prayed, and parted ways. I ached knowing that Pastor, a God-driven and God-directed man, could have been helped, and I ached for his young wife and son. Most of all, I ached for the ministry to forgotten children that would never take place.

When I saw Pastor in the hospital, he looked peaceful. At the clinic, I'd held his large hand and looked into his gentle face. He had a smile on his face, and for whatever reason, I felt deep love for the man as soon as I met him. There are few people in the world who have touched my heart and made me sing at such a deep level, but Pastor did when I realized that I could make him feel better. I should have been singing since Pastor was with the Lord, but I couldn't. The story has remained in my heart and mind, special memories that will be brought out from time to time when I need them the most.

God is in control. He is all-powerful and all-knowing. When the taxi came to take Pastor to see me, God said "no." I didn't understand how all this all fit together, but then I wasn't supposed to. I did, however, shake my head as to why God does what He does sometimes. I harbored a little anger in my soul, and I'm sure He understood. There would never be a moment when I will feel entirely myself again, but I could only conclude that Pastor's fate was God's intention.

If a person lives in the Dominican Republic, it is said that it's better for him or her to be dead than sick. For Pastor, it may have been true. I had a new fire, a new drive to have Medical Mercy make that fatalistic saying vanish for the forgotten children. Pastor had shown me the way, and maybe that's the miracle—that many would be healed because of his death

By eleven in the morning, we had a mob brewing and a crowd getting out of control. We were in a church with a lot of people coming through the doors, the team surrounded by patients. The crowd outside overwhelmed the registration process, and those with numbers began to panic and started entering the church, demanding to be seen. By then I was outside, trying to make sense of what was going on. It didn't look good, and I told someone to call the police. They arrived quickly and took control for the most part, but there was still chaos. We were witnessing firsthand the desperation of people who had nothing, needed medicines, and knew there would not likely be another chance. Could we blame them? Not really. The team was calm, and since most of them were seasoned Medical Mercy members, they knew the drill when I announced a shutdown. We got things under control and continued to see patients.

This kind of frenzy was even experienced by Jesus. A woman with a bleeding disorder had to crawl through a large crowd to touch the hem of His garment. For twelve years, she'd spent everything she had on treatments from physicians, but to no avail. Surely it was desperation that made her brave the hundreds of bodies pressing around Christ. Despite the pushing and shoving, He felt that someone had accessed His power. He turned, looking for the person responsible. When the frightened woman came forward, he didn't admonish her for creating a disturbance. He merely said, "Courage, my daughter, your faith has restored you to health" (Matthew 9:22/JB). The pupil is never above the master, and as His emissaries, we are sometimes called to walk forward into chaos, patients clamoring for attention. That's okay. They deserve it.

Marien was five years old and not a sponsored One Child Matters patient, but we saw her since it is our policy to treat the whole community in addition to sponsored children. Born at seven months gestation, she was the only surviving triplet according to her mother. The other two babies were stillborn. Marien was healthy, bright, and loveable, but here was the catch: Marien was barely breathing when she was born, causing the doctor to tell her mother, "Take this parasite home to die."

I asked the translator to repeat the phrase since I could hardly believe what the doctor had said. For a second time, all I could say was "Say it isn't so." I had to stop for a while and simply hold Marien.

These cases reminded me of the necessity of Covenant Care. When we treat patients, do we "care" while we "cure"? Indeed, do we treat the patient or just the presenting illness? If we only cure disease and ignore the broader lives of patients, we have fulfilled a contract rather than entering into a covenant to care for the entire person. This is why it's easier to plug a terminal patient into a lot of machines than to sit down with family members and discuss quality of life issues.

Pastor and Marien had received a contract. Pastor's tests hadn't been read, and Marien had received a death sentence from the doctor who delivered her. Medical services had been given, but it had been cold and unfeeling. We can contract to simply provide basic care, which is certainly necessary, or we can go beyond the immediate physical concerns that require attention and look at the person holistically, meaning that the care we give addresses body, mind, and spirit. One Child Matters strives to add a spiritual dimension to the equation so that our missions not only heal problems by using technical skills but also address a person's quality of life. When an ear infection has been cured or blood pressure medication has been prescribed, what does the person do next? Do patients return to the village and get on with life, business as usual? Or do they understand that their physical healing—their care—is part of a greater wish on His part to heal *all* aspects of their lives and give them a share in His own life.

Someone once pointed out that Jesus not only cured all who were brought to Him, but he suffered and gave everything He had to the point of death on the cross in order that we might have an all-encompassing relationship with God. Christ healed diseases of every kind, but the primal healing he gave was curing the rift between man and his creator. I think this is the deeper meaning behind the Gospel story of a paralyzed man who was brought to Jesus by lowering his stretcher through the roof of a house crowded with people. Jesus healed the man's paralysis only after addressing his spiritual condition, forgiving his sins and accepting him unconditionally. The whole person was addressed, not just paralysis.

The two kinds of healings should never be separated. They are part of a covenant relationship, and when that is lacking, medicine falls short of what it can accomplish. People are called

Fish Boy and parasites. And sometimes things go horribly wrong. They certainly did for Pastor.

They buried Pastor at the same time I examined Marien. I'd been thinking about him a great deal, and now Marien was on my mind. A life taken, a life given. One was taken by neglect, the other given as a grace from God. Still, I had to believe that the citizens of the Dominican Republic were inherently good people with good intentions, their virtues hidden under the hardship of living in poverty and abandonment. Making these trips to show the love of Christ is always a hard task. We are vulnerable, fallible, weak souls who struggle every day to do the best we can. As Second Corinthians 4:9 says, "We are persecuted but not forsaken; struck down but not destroyed" (ESV). He always gives us the courage to keep going, and He did just that in the Dominican Republic.

The Place of a Hundred Fires—that's the name of the area where we treated patients the following day. It was an area hit by fires, poverty, and crime. Two hundred thousand people lived there, isolated and struggling. We saw more of what we'd hoped *not* to see: despair and hopelessness. A sixteen-year-old girl—we believed she was really fourteen—came with her four brothers and sisters, all of whom she was caring for. Their shanty had burned down, their father had left them, and their mother worked the streets. This young girl was seven months pregnant. It was a sad case but helped explain the cycle of poverty and despair, of how such desperate conditions are perpetuated.

I also examined a six-year-old boy who reached out his hand and openly started begging. He patted my pockets and

SAY IT AIN'T SO

put out his hand, palm up. In the United States, such behavior would be frowned upon, and I can imagine a mother scolding her child for such a bold action. But this was the Dominican Republic, where people live day by day, not always sure how long they will survive. Some have outright given up. The small boy acted instinctively, imitating a behavior that was probably so prevalent that it went unnoticed. It was part of survival.

I suppose that this young child, just one among many, typified every patient we saw. They extended their arms, but not like shoppers on Black Friday trying to get the next big deal or new appliance as they run amuck through department stores. Our patients—desperate and sometimes whipped into the frenzy of a mob—prayed with open hands, petitioning God for the simple gift of His love so that they might live another day. Like me, they were saying, "Say it ain't so." I couldn't fault their prayer.

Chapter Twelve
Seeds of Hope

We went to Cambodia in late October of 2007 and flew with Mission Aviation Fellowship (MAF). We made it to Phnom Penh and checked in to the Sunway Hotel, across the street from the American Embassy. The weather was overcast, with a hard rain during the night. To get to Battambang, I flew with Paul, our MAF pilot from Australia, who was kind enough to let me do some of the flying. The ceiling was 2,000 feet, so we flew just below the clouds, Paul and I working in tandem watching the weather and the landscape, talking to each other using our cockpit resource management skills. I skirted several heavy rain cells and climbed to get over a mountain ridge, but overall it went well. I'd come a long way from controlling the ceiling fans in the living room when I was growing up.

We arrived at the clinic at Salaa Hope and oversaw members packing the medication. We had over twenty-six suitcases and rolling cargo cases of meds. We had a late dinner at the Golden Gate Hotel, our safe haven for the week. It had hot water, A/C, a bed, very slow internet, all for $12 a night. You gotta love Cambodia.

The young woman was twenty-four, shy, and quiet. She complained of headaches and menstrual cramps, but I knew there was more to what she was telling me. With a little coaxing, Chhaiden, my interpreter (and a medical student at that time), got her to tell us why she was really there: she'd been diagnosed with leukemia two years earlier and was waiting to die. She wanted to know if her death was going to be painful and if it were imminent. I looked at her and thought it was highly unlikely that she had leukemia. She was healthy, not anemic, and had lived two years with a diagnosis that kills within months in the absence of treatment.

After I questioned her further, she said she'd had a blood test that showed more white cells than red cells. She showed me the lab results which was consistent with a viral infection, but without any evidence or suspicion of leukemia. She'd been told she had leukemia and that there was nothing to be done. The diagnosis had likely been a misinterpretation of the lab values. Meanwhile, she had lived for two years, waiting for the end of her life. I assured her that she didn't have leukemia and that she would live a long time. She simply thanked me, smiled, and walked away. I watched her as she went to get vitamins and some ibuprofen for her menstrual cramps, no emotion evident in her walk or facial expression. She'd been ready for death, for she carried a letter to her mother and father, intending to have it given to them when she died. As she walked away, she tossed the letter she clutched in her hand into a trash bin, and I wondered what she'd said in the letter to her parents. On the other hand, I'm glad they won't ever have to find out, at least not for a long time, if ever.

You would think that the news I gave her—a reprieve of her death sentence—would have been joyous, but after years of waiting to die, I guess one needs time to accept that life will continue for quite a while. In fact, I think she might have been a little disappointed. Perhaps she had prepared herself for death, and now she had to look farther down the road to a life that wasn't necessarily going to be better than the fate she'd been expecting. Living in Cambodia is not for the faint of heart.

I reflected on how many other people had the same mindset. I saw despair on a regular basis, and I suspected that, for many people, a diagnosis predicting death was better than living in uncertainty from day to day. People in Cambodia lived with poverty and a shaky economy that offered few prospects for jobs. From what I'd seen in my travels, I thought it likely that hope trumped despair in most cases, but the young woman was a reminder that some lived in dark places that were hard to escape. Faith, hope, and love are powerful components of covenant care, but in the absence of hope, even the most potent medicines don't always work. Often, the arrival of a Medical Mercy team is, in itself, enough of a catalyst to generate hope in the populations we treat. But there are those who collect their medications and wander back to lives lived on the edge, and for them the best medicine we can offer is prayer that God will touch them with His light and lead them from despair.

There is never a good time to receive disturbing news.

We arrived at the village to find a swarm of people waiting for us. Within minutes, a torrential rain started, leaving us ankle deep in mud and water, with few dry places to set up examining tables, the pharmacy, registration, and spiritual counseling. We adjusted as always, and within an hour we began seeing patients. But a different kind of drama began at eleven that morning.

Kelly, our main missionary in Cambodia, was sitting in the van, cooling off and not feeling well. I checked on him and found him to be extremely pale, diaphoretic, and slightly incoherent. With backup called, a blood pressure of 80/30 was recorded, and I quickly put in a large-bore IV and ran one liter of fluid as fast as I could. We transported him to the hotel, bypassing hospitals since they were poorly staffed and equipped. At the hotel, I gave Kelly two more liters of fluid and watched him closely. By the time the team returned from seeing patients for the day, Kelly was feeling better, but he now complained of indigestion. It was clear that we had to move Kelly to a higher level of medical care, but first he needed an electrocardiogram (ECG).

The first hospital we tried sent us away, telling us they didn't have an ECG machine despite the fact that they were a trauma hospital. We drove into town and found a roadside medical clinic, where we "rescued" an old ECG machine. This primitive piece of equipment revealed significant changes in Kelly's health, and it was clear that we had to move him to Phnom Penh. At nine thirty at night, we began the four-and-a-half hour drive to Phnom Penh in torrential rain to get Kelly and his wife on an airplane for Bangkok the next day. By early morning, Kelly and his wife were on their way.

When I finally heard from Kelly, he confirmed that he'd probably had a small myocardial infarction and was scheduled for a stress test the following morning. He was doing well and in good care. Grace was with Kelly—and still is. There is always grace from Him who leads and directs us in all that we experience.

But there is another part of the story. That afternoon I saw a forty-one-year-old man who complained of a fast heart rate and a thirty-pound weight loss, telling us that these symptoms had persisted for one and two years respectively. He was extremely cachectic, anxious, and sick. His heart rate was 125 and his blood pressure was 160/110. He'd seen two doctors, both of whom acknowledged that he had heart problems but that they couldn't do anything for him since he had no money, a story that was beginning to be all too common. They told him to "go away" since he would die soon. He had no family, lived alone, and had come to us for reassurance and help. He was no different than Kelly, entitled to the best care available and an opportunity for a cure. Because he poor, however, he was denied that which is a simple right: compassion. I started him on medication and arranged for weekly follow-ups in the hope of finding a way to get him the care he needed—care that was by no means assured. I couldn't fly him to Bangkok like Kelly, and the best I could do that day was offer him grace, which was nothing more than a moment of kindness and a prescription.

Both Kelly and this man received grace, but the thing that was missing was what would happen *because* of that grace. Kelly would get better. The other man, despite grace, would more than likely die. As I watched him walk away, I saw his hand clutch the medicine he'd been given and look back just once before disappearing. I caught his eye and gave him a smile, but he looked away. The young woman waiting to die clutched a letter to her parents; the man with heart disease clutched his medication. They were so similar in all the things that really mattered. Both looked at me with no emotion since they faced death, a quick death for one, and a "living death" drawn out over a lifetime for the other. Why? They had no real hope since the game of life had been rigged in favor of those who could pony up the currency of the day. They had a contract with death rather than a covenant with life.

It is said that every turn of events in life brings you to a new place, either in location or in your heart. The two cases described above involved people with wounded hearts, and we continued to pray for them. And yet our own hearts found a new place in Cambodia, a new sense of optimism, a new realization that there are still children in this world who are innocent enough not to care about what they don't have. I saw hope in children with torn shirts, broken sandals, dirty faces, and runny noses. They smiled and were thankful that we were there. Having everything means having faith in the one who is our Father. It means having hope. I saw that in both the haves and the have-nots, and I was glad to be someone who "has." Jesus said repeatedly that we need to become like little children. Not everyone we see has hope, and that unfortunately includes children, but given their circumstances I can pass no judgment. Instead, I can only offer compassion for the difficult cases we see and refer them to a Physician who offers heroic care, and through faith I must trust that this includes hope at some point on their journey even if I can't see it or understand what form it takes. What I can be assured of is that He will not tell them to "go away."

Kelly was a reminder of this. He returned from Bangkok with good news. He'd passed all his tests and was ready to go back to work. And he shared with us the story of a woman he'd counseled one morning, a woman brimming with the ultimate hope. She asked him to pray for her personal salvation. This kind of report makes everything we do on our trips worthwhile. We do far more than dispense pills, for we fill a deeper hunger within the human spirit. The woman who prayed with Kelly had a hunger for her final destination, and it's our hope that we plant such a seed in everyone we see even if it isn't apparent at the moment.

I think of the woman with the false diagnosis of leukemia. I think of the man in need of heart care. Through our presence, maybe we planted seeds in them that will sprout later.

Seeds of hope.

Chapter Thirteen
The Palace Walls

I made an assessment trip to Ethiopia, and then it was back to Swaziland in April of 2008. I went with Teresa to see Pepe, who had been hospitalized with multi-drug-resistant tuberculosis and HIV. At twelve years old, she only weighed fourteen kilograms. Unable to take nutrition, she coughed continually, was weak, and severely withdrawn. She was also apprehensive and afraid. Having seen her a year ago, she was clearly a different child. We all wanted to do things *for* her and not *to* her. There is an end to all things, and the task is deciding when that end is. When we take extraordinary measures to extend life with technology, we're more often than not trying to make ourselves feel better, not the patient. True compassion is always other-directed.

Working in the clinic at Makholweni was difficult since we saw the impact of the epidemic of HIV and AIDS, and we encountered many cases that gave us pause, such as a fourteen-year-old boy with HIV whose grandmother had forbidden him to take his anti-retroviral medication, not believing that a fourteen year old could have HIV/AIDS. Even more troubling were the children who came without parents, looking for healthcare on their own. They had heard we were there and brought themselves to the clinic with serious complaints of illnesses that needed treatment. We gave them medications, knowing that there were no parents for them to return to. They were truly responsible for themselves, and I was amazed at their resilience and fortitude. Their survival instinct was strong, but I wondered what gave them such an indomitable will to live in the vacuum created by the absence of any family support. No child of any age should have to live without the love and nurturance of a caregiver, and such individuals are literally God's children and no one else's.

With eyes and hearts open, we traveled next to Ethiopia in July and August of 2008. Ethiopia is an African country, unique in its needs and beautiful in its own way. Behind its beauty, however, it had a large population of children with malaria, TB, malnutrition, chronic respiratory tract infections, and parasitic diseases. The children lived in single-room dwellings with sometimes ten other people, exposing them to communicable diseases. They had no running water and no toilets or sanitation, a situation that also contributed to the spread of disease.

Elyas was fourteen and came to the clinic because he'd heard that there was a team of U.S. doctors nearby. He presented with a severe body rash, scalp sores, and general malaise. He shared that his parents had died of HIV two years earlier and that his grandmother cared him for. He told us that he was taking a lot of medicines for what he thought was TB and pneumonia. He had gone to a local health clinic a year before we arrived because of sores on his leg that wouldn't heal. When he told the doctor that his parents had died of AIDS, they sent him for some tests and started him on "a lot of medicines." It was his grandmother who had told him he had pneumonia and a bad form of tuberculosis and that he would have to take medicines for a long time. If anyone asked him what was wrong, he was to tell them only what his grandmother had instilled in his mind.

He was walking down the street one day when he saw beggars holding vials of medicine in their hands; they also held slips of paper that said what they suffered from and that they were dying and needed money. Elyas recognized the vials as the same ones he'd been given and read one of the beggar's papers. It said "I have AIDS and am dying." Elyas finally knew what he had. He informed his grandmother, who nevertheless told him that he must continue to tell people that he had TB and pneumonia. Otherwise, people wouldn't want to be near him and he would end up like the beggars.

I wondered how a fourteen-year-old boy dealt with this every minute of every day of his life. He had few friends, was physically ill, and his skin was difficult to look at because of the rash and sores. He placed his trust in us, and I put him in our advanced care follow-up program so that he would be cared for every day by the One Child Matters staff in Addis Ababa. He wouldn't have to worry anymore about being shunned or dehumanized because of his disease. Elyas opened our hearts and made us realize what type of world was outside our own comfortable and familiar neighborhoods—beyond the literal walls we erect and those built of fear and discrimination.

There are still those in the United States who are stigmatized by HIV/AIDS regardless of how it has been contracted, even if the transmission occurs because of a blood transfusion. Was the grandmother really that different from anyone in the world who has a relative with the disease? The fact that she hid the disease from her own grandson was shameful, but she had compounded the problem, as well-meaning as she might have been, by isolating her son from the truth by using a wall of lies.

As the days progressed in Ethiopia, we had moments of confusion, happiness, frustration, and wonder. We saw children who were so malnourished that they didn't even measure on our growth charts. We saw people who were so dirty that their skin wasn't even visible. There were deformities, untreated injuries, and birth defects, as well as babies suckling at the breast, crying because there was no milk to be had. At Kotebe, we saw poor and isolated human beings, living day-to-day with nothing but the clothes on their backs and existing on an occasional meal of bread.

In stark contrast, the next day we met with the president of Ethiopia, exchanging "thank you's,"—us for the privilege of being in his country, and him thanking us for helping his people. The pomp and circumstance of the event was interesting at best, but for me it cemented the vast differences between the social structures of a third world country and those that frame societies in western civilization. The president of Ethiopia had heard that we were there because of the healthcare needs of an impoverished lower class, and I fervently hoped that he felt some degree of discomfort with the fact that people from another country had to travel to Ethiopia in order to care for his own citizens. After what I'd seen in the past few days, I could only speculate as to how those behind the palatial walls of Ethiopia could rest comfortably at night, knowing that just outside their gates were children dying of starvation. But I was again reminded of circumstances in the United States, where many live in mansions and gated communities only miles from the blighted, poverty-stricken areas of urban cities, and there are countless ghettos where human existence and suffering are no different than what we saw in Ethiopia.

These were difficult days. I saw the unwashed and hungry children in my mind every time I closed my eyes. And I saw the hopelessness in the eyes of those who came to the clinics, wanting more than we could possibly give them.

The last patient I saw in Bahir Dar was an old man of ninety years. He walked hunched over with a walking stick, blind and alone. A stranger had brought him to us. He sat next to me, and as I held his hand, he told me he was blind, lived on the street, had no money or family, and that he was hungry. I asked him how I could help. He looked at me through eyes that hadn't seen life in years and said quietly, "Can you help me die?" I didn't answer him. As a doctor and a human being, I didn't know how. I simply held his hand, kissed his cheek, and said a silent prayer. He was a Muslim looking to us for help. I asked the village leader who was also a pastor, if he would take care of this man and he promised he would. As I watched this old man walk away, I wondered whether I'd fallen short of what I needed to do in Ethiopia. And I wondered for a very long time if he ever got over wanting to die until one day I got a message from our facilitator in Ethiopia who told me that the village had embraced the man after we left, and he died peacefully six months later, surrounded by a community who had come to love him.

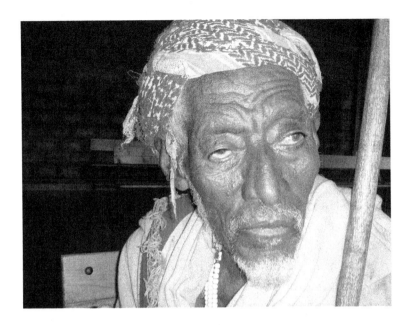

There are those who try to hide disease, and those have the courage to stare it in the face. Elyas' skin was difficult to look at, but gathering people around our clinics is a way to break down the walls we find in the third world. Jesus said, "Come to me all you who labor and are overburdened, and I will give you rest." Wherever we travel, we issue the same invitation: come. There are no barriers to God's love.

Chapter Fourteen
Fishers of Men

The first thing I felt in the Dominican Republic when we arrived in August of 2008 was the heat and the humidity, which were sticky and unrelenting. The second thing I noticed was a sense of anxiety that something was going to happen. The first feeling was real, while the second would manifest itself during our week-long stay.

We saw many different types of diseases, including parasites, flu, pneumonia, arthritis, breast cancer, HIV, and just plain old age. We perceived an unrelenting need from the people we treated to just be heard. It sounds simple enough, but with hundreds of patients waiting to be seen, the oppressive heat taking its toll on us, and the pharmacy running out of medicines, it was a difficult task.

A four-year-old boy, mentally handicapped, was brought to us by his father, also mentally handicapped, and he was the child's only caretaker. He only wanted to know if he was doing a good job taking care of his little boy, a simple but heartfelt inquiry that's lacking in even affluent, developed countries among those who have no mental handicap at all. We also saw a little girl who was born with her intestines hanging out. The local physicians had told the mother that they could do nothing until the child was much older. The family had lived with this condition every day—living on the edge, waiting for the loops of the girl's intestines to twist and get infected even though the problem could easily have been fixed at birth. There was not much to do for these two patients other than to listen, and it was like that for most of the people who showed up at the clinics. Others complained of cough and cold, but the reality was that all they wanted was to have someone tell them they were well. We did that over and over again, almost 2,000 times, with smiles on our faces and love in our hearts.

On the very last day, however, we saw a patient who was having a severe anaphylactic reaction. His airway began to close, his eyes swelled shut, and he was rapidly deteriorating. We ran an IV, Benadryl and Albuterol were administered, and an epi-pen was thrust into his thigh. Without any of these interventions, he would have died. After we caught our breath, we wondered why these particular people had come to us. From an even larger perspective, we wondered why *anyone* in *any* country showed up. We knew, of course, the superficial answer: they needed medical treatment. But was there a deeper reason that our patients had come to the clinics, and had the individuals been prompted by something greater than the fact that they'd heard that U.S. doctors were in the vicinity? Had a larger hand touched their minds and spirits to seek us out for prayer, medical, treatment, and attention?

Two possibilities came to mind. Jesus chose His first disciples when walking by the shore of the Sea of Galilee, asking them to put out into the deep despite Peter's protestation that they'd already been on the water all night, catching nothing. Without understanding the request, Peter obeyed. Miraculously, they netted a catch that filled two boats to the point of almost sinking. The fish were suddenly just there. After returning to shore, Jesus told his first disciples that from then on they would become fishers of men. I and my team don't always understand why we have been summoned to do certain tasks in various countries, but we obey His will without trying to reason everything out. We have been called to be fishers of men.

Later in his ministry, Jesus preached to thousands in the countryside of Palestine. There were no fliers, no PR. People came to hear his words and to be healed. He showed up, and they were simply there, called by the Spirit to hear the preaching of God made flesh. I can only conclude that the Spirit draws certain people to us for His inscrutable purposes. We put out into deep water, and people flock to us for prayer and healing. Other times they just want to be seen and heard.

I find it interesting that the needs of many of those who flocked to Jesus had diseases that were obvious to anyone looking at them, and yet Jesus frequently—and curiously—asked them "What do you want me to do for you?" (Mark 10:51/ JB). If a blind man approached, Jesus certainly knew why the man was there, but He asked the question anyway. He traveled to towns and villages, and people were suddenly there. Jesus wanted to hear what was on their minds, wanted for them to speak and make known their needs. Sometimes they just wanted to be in His presence or receive encouragement, wisdom, and advice.

This is what I'd sensed at the beginning of the trip—that people were going to show up in order to be heard. Our primary goal this time was to be present to them, to open our hearts and ears and listen to their questions and complaints, praying with them and giving them reassurance in addition to medicine. This, therefore, was my third "feeling" on the trip. Our job each time is to put out into deep water and lower our nets. We have seldom failed to receive a catch filled to overflowing.

As to the fish we net—the individuals He draws to us—God is in the front office managing the details. We're servants out on the lake doing His bidding. We show up with medicine, and He fills out the spiritual paperwork.

That's what it's like when you sail deep waters.

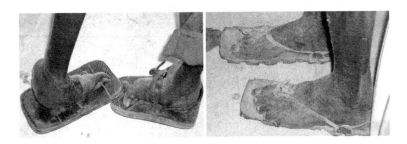

Chapter Fifteen

The Fall of a Sparrow

We arrived in Kenya in October of 2008, sliding into the country under an early morning fog. Our hotel rooms weren't ready, but the sun came out and burned away the fog. Things always have a way of balancing out on these trips, plus they're a reminder that we can expect the good and the bad, the miracle and the heartbreak, resistance and cooperation. After finally getting settled in our hotel, we sorted over 5,000 doses of prescriptions side by side with World Health—stuffing baggies and then labeling and packing them. Sometimes it's the little things that are required of us. That's okay, too. The person who is faithful in small things can be entrusted to be faithful with the large.

Lokori is a very small village south of Lake Turkana, isolated and very remote. When we visited, it served as the base for Pastor Park and his wife, who ran a ministry for One Child Matters children in six villages within a thirty-two kilometer area surrounding Lokori, and we visited many of them over the next four days. There was nothing in Lokori to make it stand out except the people. A dirt strip was used by MAF to land there, but it was a ten-hour drive to the nearest civilized town.

There was no electricity, water—nothing. The area was potentially dangerous, with bandits who preyed on the vulnerable, and for that reason we had two armed guards with us the whole time we remained in the region.

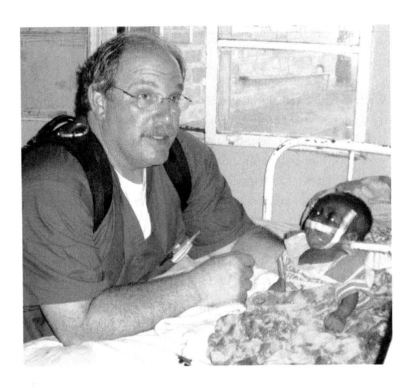

A three-month-old baby girl, Emma, was brought to us by her mother. The mother had no breast milk, and the baby weighed less than five pounds. She was minimally responsive, extremely dehydrated, and grunted with respiratory difficulty. I cut some IV tubing and placed it down her nose as an NG (nasogastric) tube, and we fed her oral rehydration salts (ORS) since she couldn't suck. Given her poor condition, we decided to take her to a local clinic, where we did an old-fashioned blood smear to check for malaria. There was none. The nurse who ran the clinic found some old IV catheters, and I placed one in Emma's hand. We also found some IV antibiotics, which we gave her. Emma stayed the night in order to get more NG feedings. All in all, it was a very difficult day. We are commanded to care for the least among us, and Emma represented the smallest and most helpless of His children

The next day, we got to the village of Lokwii after a fifteen-minute ride into the bush. Lokwii is a small isolated village in the middle of nowhere, and we set up our medical clinic in a church Pastor Park had built. We saw 300 children and walked through the village at lunch and saw how they lived, receiving a goat and a rooster as gifts. I wasn't sure sure what to do with them (we gave them to Pastor Park), but it gave a whole new meaning to medical insurance and co-pays.

We checked on little Emma and saw that she was a little better, but we still couldn't find any formula. She was weak, and we were getting tired and feeling very vulnerable as we beheld her small face. Could we do anything that would make a difference for the baby? Just how far should we go? The ethics of third world medicine were hitting home: do what you can with what you have, and do it the best way you can. No more, no less. We all sensed that Emma would die despite this ethic, but our hearts were reluctant to let her go.

And that is what happened. Emma died. She stopped breathing the following afternoon while we tended to other patients. Medically, we'd simply run out of time. The health center's director visited us at Pastor Park's house and informed us of Emma' death. A picture taken twenty-four hours earlier indicated that maybe she might make it, but it wasn't to be.

Christ was summoned by a synagogue official named

Jarius, whose twelve-year-old daughter was dying. When Jesus arrived, the girl had died, although He said she was only sleeping before bringing her back to life a few minutes later. But such a joyful scenario didn't play out for Emma. As was the case with Pastor, God had said "no."

Another verse came to mind, however, one that seemed appropriate for the situation. Jesus told His followers that not a single sparrow falls to the ground without the Father's permission. Our Father in heaven is a god of the fallen sparrow, and Emma was surely a tiny sparrow who had been called home. Despite our heartache, it is not for us to question when it is time for anyone to return to Him, whether it is a baby named Emma or a ninety-year-old man in Ethiopia who longs for death but cannot find it. Psalm 139 says that God knows the number of our days even before we are born. There is a master plan that we are not privy to, but that notwithstanding, I do not think God minded when we shed tears for a sparrow who lived three months and no longer. Jesus wept when he heard that his friend Lazarus had died, which tells us that God knows of our grief. For reasons we cannot understand, He sometimes allows our hearts to break. But I wonder if Emma accomplished a very important mission in her brief time on earth, one that was as important as any achieved by someone who lives a very long life. Perhaps her purpose was precisely to make us shed tears and forever keep her image in our minds. Maybe God wanted her to teach us how important all the sparrows are in the countries we visit. We already knew their importance, but it is conceivable that once in a while we need a more specific reminder in the form of the most humble and innocent, such as a baby named Emma.

This is only speculation, but I do know that we will remember her. Even when a baby lives only a matter of weeks or months, we must still give thanks. All lives are gifts, and all have meaning. I am confident that Emma did her Father's will.

We went farther into the bush, crossing rivers and using a four-wheel drive the whole way. The Land Cruiser was packed high with medication. One of the last children we saw had severe conjunctivitis and a high fever. Oral antibiotics, Paracetamol, and oral fluids were all that we had to offer. In the United States she would have been admitted to the hospital for IV therapy, but once again we did the best we could with what we had.

We'd been around the bush and seen a lot of cases that we could only have imagined seeing before we got there. We began to realize that we had been given a rare opportunity to witness life at a different level, but we struggled to assimilate this realization into our lives. Would it change our perspectives, goals, and values? We asked these questions of ourselves, waiting for the answers to appear.

Faith, of course, is more than just the moment of conversion. It is a journey to deeper levels of understanding. Jesus once healed a blind man, whose first report was that he could see, but that the people he saw looked like trees walking around. When Jesus touched the man's eyes a second time, his cloudy vision was healed and he saw clearly—saw at a different level. I think that was what happened to us in the bush. Indeed, I believe it happens on all of our trips. We are continually touched by Him, enabling us to see deeper into the hearts and minds of our patients and into the heart of the third world itself. In turn, we see Christ more clearly as well, standing in the bush or Gaza or Garbage City.

We had been changed in Kenya. Our vision was sharper, and we had once more received grace to help us along our journey to encounter Him in the names and faces and people we met. We could even see His hand in the fall of a sparrow.

Chapter Sixteen

Smiles and a Cup of Cold Water

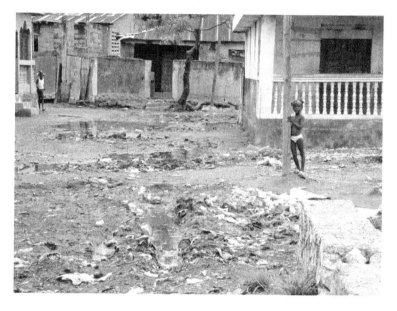

I made an assessment of the children in Haiti in April of 2009 in preparation for our medical team trip scheduled for the end of October. I'd been to some poor countries, but this one seemed to stand out a little bit more since it is the poorest in the western hemisphere. The reason for its status is simple: isolation. Due to political turmoil, bad publicity, violence, and uprisings, Haiti suffers from a sense of extreme isolationism, somewhat self-imposed, that prevents many people on the outside from entering, let alone from understanding its dire poverty. One Child Matters had taken on 1,000 children in ten projects, and all but two were isolated, wilderness-confined, and poor beyond poor. The children, for the most part, had the usual maladies, degrees of malnutrition, and a sense of longing that accompanies profound need. Their faces were either bright and happy, or empty and drawn. I'd seen this kind of dynamic before, and Haiti presented such stark contrasts precisely because of its poverty and isolationism. Hope and despondency are strange bedfellows, but I understood all too well how they could coexist in such a climate of need and suffering.

I visited the Justinian Hospital, which had a pediatric residency program, and saw a baby dying in front of my eyes. I gave the staff a quick bedside lecture on resuscitation, and within a few hours the baby had some life in him. I decided to use the hospital as a referral for the sickest children we would see on our coming trip.

Haiti is filled with dirt, pollution, and filth, a dark filter that made it difficult to see the lives underneath. I sensed that we would need to pick through all of it in order to find the clean hearts of those who know to whom they belong. All 1,000 of the children that we'd see were reaching out, and I couldn't wait to hear their hearts sing when we returned.

Our team of almost fifty—doctors, nurses, missionaries, and interpreters—made it to the Dominican Republic with over 600 pounds of medicine. We had a short glitch at customs, but our paperwork helped, and after discussion, negotiation, and persistence, we made it through. The team was ready, and the following day we were bound for Haiti. We had a three-hour drive to the border, and as the scenery and atmosphere changed, so did our mood as we grew somber and worried. What were we in for?

We arrived on the Dominican Republic side of the border, and a bridge was waiting for us. The bridge spanned the Dajabón River, nicknamed Massacre River for the killing of thirty Frenchman by Spanish settlers in 1728 (and later for the atrocities that occurred during the Parsley Massacre genocide of 1937 under the regime of Dominican President Rafael Trujillo). Thousands upon thousands were butchered and violated. We crossed the border with all of the medicine, headed for a barren and desolate land. Haiti customs and passport control awaited us, but our paperwork and contacts held and we got through. Nothing was confiscated, and there were no entrance fees—only a few bribes, which we had expected. We picked up two prearranged plain clothes armed policemen who would be with us for the week, and they helped us make it through additional customs and roadblocks—and another bribery request. Without our escorts we would have been in some serious trouble with the "officials." In Haiti, it paid to have people who knew the ropes and had some firepower on their belts. We made it to Cap-Haitien, which can only be described as pummeled by poverty, garbage, isolation, war, and corruption. We arrived at our hotel, and on the following day we finally started that for which we had come: seeing patients.

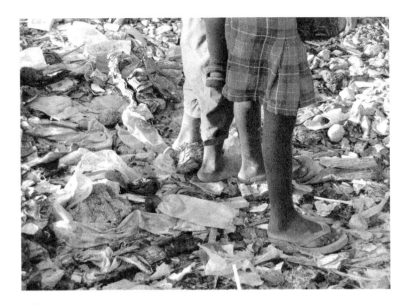

During the first two days, we had to negotiate bad roads, potholes, people, animals, narrow streets, and garbage—there was garbage everywhere—and it was hot and humid. We didn't see anything out of the ordinary—rashes, pneumonia, urinary tract infections, and the like—and also played with the children, who did the "chicken dance."

Given the extreme filth and garbage, I brought a small water filtration system that worked amazingly well. Using a five-gallon bucket, I drilled a hole in the side, attached a pipe connector and a small filter to allow the dirty water to drain using gravity. The water came out crystal clear, and with a crowd around me, I drank it. With a $45 filter kit, we had pure drinking water for an entire village. It might seem like a small thing, especially in countries where one simply turns a tap, but to the very poor, clean water is a luxury as well as a major way to help eliminate disease and parasites.

One of our doctors saw an eighty-year-old woman who'd had a stroke the year before, and one side of her body was paralyzed as a result, which naturally included one side of her face. When asked what we could do for her, she said, "Can you help me smile again?" Like clean water, we take for granted something as simple as the ability to move our limbs or facial muscles, but in the poorest nation in the hemisphere, nothing could be taken for granted. We saw many smiles on our trips, smiles from people happy to receive decent medical treatment, but in this case the request was to be able to smile in the first place. I wish we could have granted the woman's wish, but maybe we left her with an inner smile. Sometimes that's the best we can hope for. Either way, it reminded us to be thankful for everything—each breath of air, each blink of an eye, each step we take. For so many people in the world, these things are treasures beyond reach.

Fortunately, we saw smiles on the faces of many children, which was a miracle since Haiti was a torn country devastated by war, revolts, corruption, and poverty. It is said that "You're lucky to be alive in Haiti," but the smiles on the children we saw as they danced and played with the team seemed to make up for that. The smile of a child is richer than all of the gold in world. We smiled all the way back to the hotel that night, and I fell asleep with a smile on my face. Who knows? We couldn't give the old woman a smile, but maybe we gave the children a few smiles they otherwise wouldn't have shown. Even if we'd managed to give nothing else despite the arduous journey to Haiti and the frustrating border crossing, the smiles would have made it worthwhile. We are told in scripture that we will not lose our reward if we give a cup of cold water to one of the little ones—and the water filtration accomplished that—but I think that a smile will gain a reward as well. Both give life and nourish the spirit.

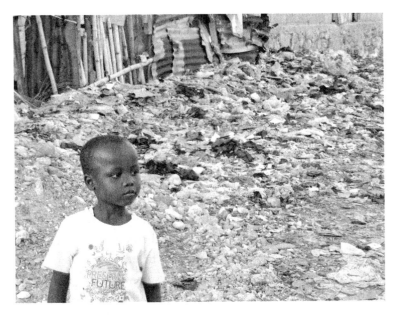

A woman came to the clinic carrying a limp child, about one and a half years old, with a large head and cerebral palsy. She'd found the child the day before in a pile of garbage on the street. We rushed the child to the back room and started IV fluids and antibiotics, and he looked better in a relatively short time. The local doctor left to find an orphanage that was willing to take the child, but he and I suspected something wasn't quite right. The way the woman held the child, looked at him, and got him to eat spoke volumes. I got an interpreter to help understand the events of the previous day. Where had she found this child? Had she ever seen him before? Did she have any idea who the mother could be? I found out that she had ten children and lived on the street. The local doctor returned to say that the orphanage was full and that this child with cerebral palsy would be too difficult to care for anyway.

We talked about our suspicion regarding who the child really belonged to and then spoke with the mother again. We told her that we would help her and "her" child. She thanked us, and we all knew what the real story was now. We gave her the opportunity to say what she herself could not. We didn't shame, judge, or humiliate her. She had tried to find a way to procure care for the child beyond what she could provide herself to the point of giving him up, but she hadn't been able to openly tell us the truth. We got the local pastor to bring her into his church and set up continuing medical care for her son with the local doctor. We also got the child started on a nutrition program and gave him much needed medicines. The woman left with the child as she had come: a mother.

In a world such as ours, with poverty and hardship beyond description, people do desperate things. We gave the mother a sense of dignity, and the child would have a chance at life. How good that life would be was something only time would tell. Dignity and a chance at life: that was the cup of cold water we had to offer these children of God.

I asked the question over and over again: for what purpose were we there? After our experience with the mother and child, it became even clearer. We were present to serve those who had nothing, who out of desperation would give up their own children to ensure they would have better lives. We were there to give hope, and whenever possible, smiles and a cup of cold water.

Another day in Haiti. Events at the clinic weren't that unusual, but the road was so bad that we had to park the bus several blocks away and walk due to the ruts and the water. We saw what no one should ever have to behold. Nobody should have to live in the filth we were surrounded by—and we had visited many countries where filth was abundant, such as Cairo. No child should have to play in the garbage, but then again, who were we to judge when we came from a neatly manicured, sanitized world? We had options and lifestyles that didn't revolve around day-to-day survival. Garbage was collected, houses were cleaned, lawns were mowed, and in most areas there was an emergency care clinic or pharmacy within walking or driving distance of our homes. If people had been born into a completely different world than I was, I couldn't look at them with anything but sorrow and compassion. Filth and garbage were all they knew and all they had to work with. I couldn't help but wonder if I could live in a place like that after a lifetime of privilege. I'd like to think I could—that I could answer any call—but the truth is that I just wasn't sure. I could only hope that, with His grace, I was up to any task He gave me.

When I looked back at the week, I saw that the team had been changed as usual. Who we are on the first day of a trip is not who we are on the last day. This time, we realized that life passes by too quickly, and if we don't slow down we'll run out of time to experience all that has been given to us, for we are blessed in ways that most of the world's population isn't. We have smiles, and we also have that cup of cold water whenever we need it. We also have family support, unlike the mother of ten.

I realized that the hard task was not to forget these lessons once we returned home, lessons about the simple things in life. But time—that, too, is a gift, and one day it will run out. A man who had a near-death experience saw, in classic fashion, his whole life passing before his eyes, as if watching a movie. His reflection was this: every one of us will watch the movie that was our lives. We should make sure that it's a movie worth watching.

I think we made a difference in Haiti. One day I will again see the faces of the children and adults we treated there. Indeed, the people we see on all of our trips will be part of my own movie. As long as it contains smiles and cups of cold water, I'm confident it will be a movie worth watching.

Chapter Seventeen

There but for the Grace of God

The damage was horrific. The epicenter of the earthquake that hit Haiti on January 12, 2010 was in the town of Léogane, approximately sixteen miles west of Port-au-Prince. Three million people were affected, and with over a quarter million homes destroyed or rendered unlivable, people lived on the street and in shantytowns that appeared overnight. The estimate for the number killed ranged from 100,000 to 220,000, but it was hard to know the exact figure with chaos compromising reliable intelligence from the countryside. Bodies were collected and buried in mass graves, and with fifty-two aftershocks during the following month, conditions only grew worse. Our One Child Matters director in Haiti said that the projects in the northern part of the country had not sustained much damage, but that Port-au-Prince was a total disaster. Medical Mercy, therefore, was going back to Haiti. We'd seen the filth and the garbage of the country just a few months earlier, but with such tremendous damage to an already shaky infrastructure, and with homes that were not constructed according to any real building code, we anticipated that we would see devastation on a new scale.

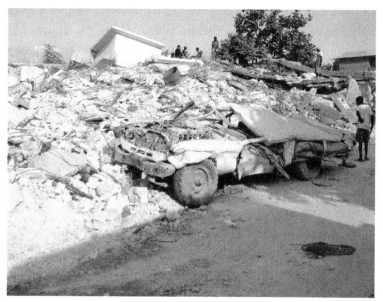

Medical Mercy had been a longtime partner with Mission of Hope Haiti, which had a clinic only a few miles from Port-au-Prince. A medical team was present and had been working nonstop for two days after the quake. Our initial plan was to either relieve or assist the team already there. After endless telephone calls, emails, and pulling in some favors, I contacted medical team members and formed a tentative plan to leave for Haiti via charter jet within seventy-two hours following the quake. We anticipated working near Port-au-Prince for a week, although there was a lot of civil unrest in the country, and with the charter not a done deal, we knew that we might have to cancel at the last minute. Assuming the final pieces fell into place, it was going to be a risky mission, far from anything we had done before, but the team members I'd assembled, all seasoned, were willing to accept the uncertainty that accompanied such disaster relief and to follow where He pointed.

We hooked up with a chartered 737 out of Miami that was

destined for Port-au-Prince, one we would share with a host of other relief organizations. But the cargo hold of the charity 737 was going to be so full that we would have to carry our suitcases on board, which meant taking them through TSA security. Our hope was that TSA would let us through due to our medical mission relief status, although the agency was known for its arbitrary treatment of travelers. The entire time we prepared, we watched the news, and the reports from the ground in Haiti were more than a bit unsettling. Plus we were going to a place less fortunate with heavy hearts and spirits, but if we could offer encouragement and grace with a smile, we knew this new kind of mission was something that God would direct.

We managed to get our entire luggage on board—a small gift from God—and 5,000 pounds of supplies, much of it ours, was loaded into the cargo bay. We arrived on the island, and the airport at Port-au-Prince was chaos. We parked on the tarmac among C-130s, helicopters, and private jets, all crowded together like people on a morning subway. We unloaded our cargo and waited on the tarmac for our ride, which eventually came and took us to our base. An hour and a half later we arrived at our camp, passing a mass grave with thousands of passed bodies. The bodies were piled under bright lights, bulldozers moving them about without feeling. The smell was horrid. Our first hours there were a grim reminder of the scale of tragedy and devastation.

The reminders kept coming. We met other personnel at the base: a group of doctors who were working in hospitals and providing on-the-fly post-op care; and an ob-gyn doc who performed an emergency C-section without anesthesia, losing both mother and baby. The crisis in Haiti had a lot in common with my days in Cambodia in 1980, where harsh decisions had to be made, resulting in a great deal of neglect, suffering, and death.

We went to bed and rose early due to an aftershock. Everything rumbled and shook, and we ran outside and saw that the building we were staying in hadn't sustained any damage. Still, we wondered how safe the coming days would be if the island continued to experience tremors, and I decided to sleep outside from then on. Each passing hour reinforced that we were in new territory when it came to conducting a mission to provide relief to a hurting region.

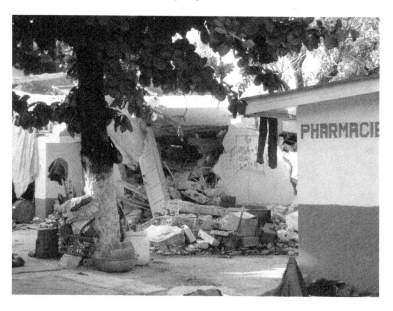

We drove to Carrefour, a poor community in Port-au-Prince, and set up a field unit at the end of a small street surrounded by collapsed buildings and the smell of rotting bodies. Just 300 yards from us a person was pulled from the rubble, which was a measure of how close we were to what people were seeing on their televisions on the six o'clock news. We saw a great deal of trauma: fractured femurs, ankles, arms, legs, as well as lacerations, concussions, and a comatose woman. Two babies, both under twenty-four days old, were brought in for severe dehydration. The mothers hadn't eaten since the earthquake and had no breast milk left. We placed an IV in each baby and ran solutions. One baby recovered, while the other remained marginal as we left.

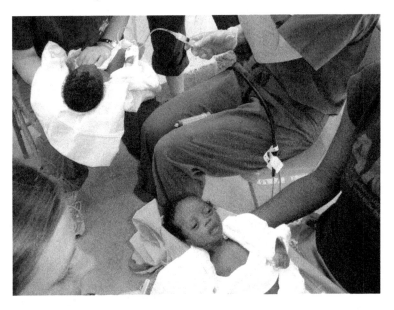

The look in people's eyes, the smells, and the atmosphere—it could only be felt on the ground, not through a television screen with images edited to fit a five-minute slot on the news. The look of despair and hurt on a single face said more than a thousand-page book. There's an old saying that "There but for the grace of God go you and I." It could have been any one of us wandering the Haitian streets or trapped by debris, but the people of Haiti had been in the wrong place at the wrong time, and they were the ones paying the price for a natural disaster that came to a country already oppressed in so many ways. Children and adults had amputated arms and legs, large lacerations, and crushing injuries. Especially haunting were the blank looks on the faces of those we served. Next to us was the destruction of buildings, homes, roads, and lives. We were left with the usual question of "Why did it have to happen at all?" It seemed that the question always returned in the face of tragedies that were worse than the ones we'd seen before, but our immediate task was not to seek an answer, only to place casts, suture, debride wounds, clean abrasions, give IV fluids, and pray.

The boy was ten years old. As I dressed his amputated left arm, he winced only once and turned his head away, afraid to show emotion. He had lain under the rubble of his house for three days while his mother lay on his shattered left arm. He said she died on the second day. I bandaged his arm, hugged him, and watched as he walked away, cared for by a neighbor. His father and two siblings had yet to be found. He had no tears, no emotion. It was obvious that the mental trauma of the population would be as severe as the physical wounds they'd sustained. (Members of our own team, in fact, suffered from mild forms of PTSD when we arrived home.)

One of the twenty-four-day-old babies that we had cared for was brought back. His mother said that she couldn't care for him any longer and asked us to look after him. We placed him in an orphanage, and that would be his home from then on, a legacy that would follow him forever. The mother came back the next day and followed us around. The baby had been her first child, and it was obvious that she couldn't come to grips with her decision, but then that was the case with tens of thousands of people. Blank faces, empty eyes. What do you do when the very ground you stand on forsakes you?

We arrived at a local hospital destroyed by the quake. The only thing left standing was the outpatient clinic. The courtyard, littered with rubble, was filled with patients and families living under tarps and sheets, all waiting for help. Seven days after the quake, there hadn't been any food or emergency medical care for these people, although two young Haitian doctors and a few nurses had spent several days doing the best they could with the little they had. We set up a makeshift clinic and saw over 300 patients in five hours. The hospital had a sign that identified it as a public hospital. The sign had FOOD FOR THE POOR on it as well. It was a beacon, the light of which had been extinguished.

The homes and buildings that had been destroyed next to our field site in Carrefour continued to be cleared of rubble. The smell of the dead within was strong, and as I watched the large bucket of the bulldozer lift tons of concrete, I saw the corner of a dress flutter. I turned away, not wanting to see the full picture.

On our last day, we had time to play with some of the children, singing, dancing, and sharing the crackers and cookies we had brought with us. They smiled, laughed, and danced, but a few days earlier they had been frightened, wondering if they had any future at all. That night, they would sleep in the street again, afraid to go indoors because of the tremors. It was refreshing to see their smiles, and for a brief moment they forgot the events of recent days and became children again.

I sat with many victims of the quake and heard them ask questions, the same ones I asked myself. They told me they would wait for answers as to why this happened and what would become of them. I looked for answers as well. There would never be a concrete answer, and I could only wish that the hearts of those who lived though the Haiti earthquake—those who lost whole families—would someday find understanding and live lives that were rich in love and grace. We came here to find a way to help, and in a very small way, we did.

Chapter Eighteen
Slums and Rag Pickers

I was in London awaiting my flight to New Delhi to make an assessment of a planned Medical Mercy trip to India in April of 2010. It had only been one week since I'd returned from Haiti, and the sights and sounds and patients I'd encountered were still in the forefront of my mind. One doesn't walk away from a disaster of such magnitude without an indelible imprint on one's soul, and we planned to return to the country at some future point. Haiti would be trying to heal for years to come.

But there were other places with people in great need, places that God called us to visit so that we might be His presence, and India was one of those countries to which He was directing us. India had thousands of abandoned and forgotten children that One Child Matters was responsible for, and Medical Mercy would assume the daunting task of taking a team there to care for over thousands of children. I expected to see squalor, filth, poverty, and suffering, and I wasn't so sure that it would be qualitatively different from what I'd seen in Haiti. The landscape might be different, but the human heart seems to be the same wherever I go.

So I continued my journey, my heart still heavy from Haiti, and I expected it to be so for a very long time. India, Cambodia, Swaziland, Egypt, Mozambique, and all the countries we go to weighed heavy on my heart. I kept close to me a Latin phrase: "After the shadows I await the light." I hoped that it would come soon.

Sangam Vihar is considered one of the largest unauthorized colonies of Asia and has a population close to two million. This slum area had in it a subdivision of a slum, as hard as that is to imagine, called the Rag Picker slum, and that is where One Child Matters was located. The Rag Picker slum was only one of the many sub-slums within the large Sangam Vihar colony, and when I visited, the populations was about 200,000 people, all of whom were rag pickers, meaning that they were garbage collectors, though not the kind of salaried workers one envisions in the United States. It had a striking resemblance to Garbage City in Cairo. There was no potable water, no toilets, and no sewage. Dwellings were made of plastic or other material found in piles of garbage. People went to the city every morning to collect garbage that they later sorted through to recycle, though again, this kind of recycling bore no resemblance to recycling in the U.S. Workers made about one dollar a day doing this. Most children were not allowed to go to school because they were needed to pick through the garbage in order to sustain the family.

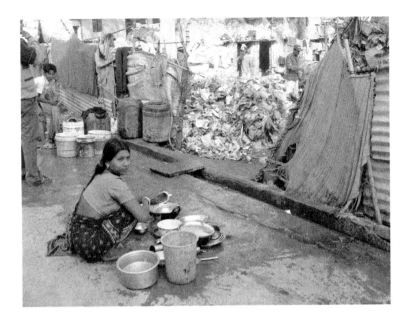

Families lived on small parcels of land owned by wealthy individuals who rented the area, a bizarre take on the medieval feudal system. The property was usually small, no larger than a sixteenth of an acre, and rented for about $300 a month, which was split among the families living there. There was a middleman, or contractor, who was hired by the owner of the property. He collected the sorted garbage, paid twenty-five to fifty cents cents for a bag of plastic, and then turned around and sold it for five to six dollars, giving the owner a cut. The rag pickers were essentially slaves.

In such a dirty and merciless system, it wasn't surprising that twenty percent of the children didn't see their fifth birthday due to the illnesses they contracted living in the squalor. One Child Matters was there to pave the way to a better life for these children by first and foremost bringing them medical care. Pastor Koshy and his wife Joicy had been there for fourteen years and had a remarkable educational, nutritional, and spiritual program going with help from One Child Matters. It was our hope to augment their efforts through our clinic work.

Kalkaji is situated in the southern area of New Delhi and is one of the city's largest slums. The population was around 150,000, of which 40,000 were children under the age of fourteen. It was known for its high drug addiction rate and gang-related activities. Almost all of the Kalkaji dwellers were illiterate, people of the labor class who earned less than two dollars a day, assuming they worked at all. Since most of the men were either drug addicts or alcoholics, the money they made went to feeding their addictions, leaving nothing for the family. Many of the women worked as servants in nearby houses while the children stayed home to care for their younger siblings. Sometimes the girls were sold by their parents to gang-like sex traffickers in order to get money to live on.

The slum area had no water facilities, and the children had to carry water in buckets from water trucks that arrived in the slum on rare occasions. With few children attending school, they fell prey to cycles of illiteracy and poverty, never leaving the slum area as they grew older. The rooms they occupied were no bigger than five feet by eight feet, with as many as nine people living in these confined spaces. There were no toilet facilities except for a small communal area that had a line with a two-hour wait to use the bathroom. It was easier and quicker to use the alleyways instead. The sanitation situation, therefore, was ideal for breeding disease.

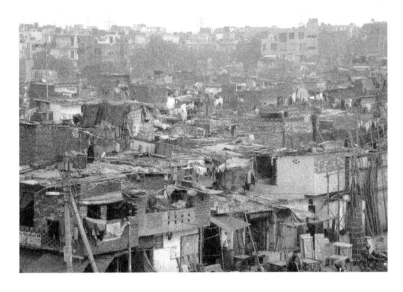

∽◊∾

The slum of Rum Nagar was an hour and a half south of New Delhi. It was one of the biggest slums of Faridabad, and was located near the Faridabad Thermal Power Station, which was directly behind the New Town Railway Station. Around 50,000 families lived in this area in sub-human conditions. These individuals were migrants from Bihar, Uttar Pradesh, and Rajasthan. Most were daily laborers in the powerhouse or other factories. Some were rickshaw pullers and rag pickers. The slum had a big town dump, and many children between the ages of four and seventeen worked in the area—they, too, picked through items to be recycled—which contained toxic material from various factories in Faridabad.

There was opposition from dump yard gangs and Hindu fundamentalist groups, both of which had damaged the property of a nearby school where children went to learn and eat.

I visited the school, which was on the very edge of the slum, but I was advised not to go any farther into the slum itself. It was currently under review as to whether or not we could go there to hold a medical clinic due to the resistance of the gangs and fundamentalists. The children there were not as healthy as I had seen elsewhere, and there had been reported instances of child kidnappings.

I'd been right. These areas were every bit as filthy as the poorest sections of Haiti. In fact, garbage had been turned into a marketable commodity. Recycling is all well and good, but not when it deprives children of an education and exposes them to disease and toxic waste. They belonged in school, but instead were subjected to hard labor, illness, and sex trafficking. These people were literal and figurative slaves, owned and used by wealthy people to make money from garbage.

When I was told that I could not go deep into the heart of the slums, I was reminded of the time Jesus traveled to the region of the Gadarenes, a section of which was avoided by travelers since two men were chained to a tomb there. Wild and fierce, they were possessed by demons and often broke their bonds, screaming as they roamed about naked. There was no real solution to their plight since no one in the local community could control them.

There were sections in these Indian slums that were also to be avoided, dangerous areas where gangs and rag pickers and their masters made it unsafe to travel. In a real sense, I think these areas—and many like them around the world—harbored unclean spirits that we must fight with prayer assuming we're allowed in at all. For the Gadarene demoniacs, only Jesus could drive out their demons and restore them to normalcy. Once again, He demonstrated heroic care and a covenant relationship, mindful not only of physical disease but the darkness that plagued certain people and regions. Our teams had engaged in spiritual warfare before, and I had no doubt that a great deal of prayer would be required to enter these slums and treat the forgotten children.

We had other places to visit first, but the slums weighed heavily on my mind, as did the devastation in Haiti. Was there an end to the poverty, crime, drugs, and neglect? I could only shake my head and wonder.

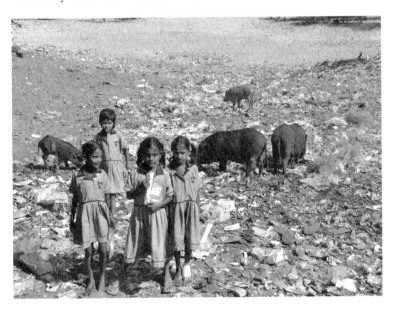

Chapter Nineteen

Discernment

I did a lot of thinking on my way back from India. Slums and poverty were the mainstay of the assessment, with medical needs not drastically different from what we were accustomed to seeing in many other countries: malnutrition, worms, rashes, chronic pneumonias, tuberculosis, and vitamin deficiency. One would think that after all the countries we'd visited that we would find it easy to go through our setup and protocols since the diseases are essentially the same and the living environments are not that much different from place to place. What is different from country to country, however, is the people—who they are and how they cope, or why they live the way they do as they try to find a better way of life. It's the interaction we have with those we serve that reminds us that each culture, each person, and each community is different. The antibiotics we administer are the same regardless of where we are, but the people who seek them are unique.

But shouldn't we be gracious to all regardless of their living situations? Of course. Does compassion change from one culture to the next? No, it shouldn't, but I realized that our understanding of the manner in which people lived needed to change. Without that understanding, we miss the most important part of a covenant relationship with those who come to us, which involves trust, acceptance, and honesty. We start to assume that we know what is best for those who are less fortunate, and we are often far from being right. Intentionally or not, we put our own value systems into place based on our own lives and circumstances. The result is that sometimes we make decisions for others that may leave them worse off than they were before. I came to this conclusion because of what I'd seen when trying to make lives better for the less fortunate. Often they were very happy with what they had, and putting them in a different place other than that to which they were accustomed had the potential to cause them angst and confusion. That was the case with the two lifelong friends in Garbage City. I'd tried to impose my value system on people whose contentment was alien to me.

My parents and grandparents were from Egypt and Syria. My parents emigrated to the United States, and I vividly remember traveling to Egypt with my father to get our extended family from Egypt to the States so that they could live a better life. My great uncle, my grandfather's brother, was eighty years old when we got him to the U.S. He lived in San Francisco for the remaining years of his life, but always living on Egypt time by keeping his watch set to what time it was in Cairo. He was heartbroken at being transplanted and missed his life and country. He may have been less fortunate in Egypt, but I believe we compromised the last few years of his life by trying to give him a better life than what he had previously known. Less fortunate? By whose standard? I'm not suggesting that those who live in the slums should be encouraged to stay there, or that it's up to us to move them and give them what we regard as better. What I *am* suggesting is that we need to understand that the lives they have, even though they are hard and difficult are, in fact, their lives and no one else's. We should make them better by helping them within their own community, making their lives a little better right where they are. The simple things in life can make all the difference in the world—clean water, toilets, and electricity—but people should be surrounded by those they know in a country they love. That's what will touch their spirits, and if we ignore their inner life, then we miss the point of helping them to begin with.

Jesus related to people according to who they were and where they lived. He ministered in the homes of tax collectors, occasionally dining with rich members of the Jewish Sanhedrin, but he also related to the people who flocked to him in the countryside, people who experienced great suffering and physical handicaps. And before His ascension into heaven, he instructed his apostles to go forth into the world to spread His message—the world, with its diverse cultures and populations.

That is the mission of Medical Mercy: to go into the world, not to bring the world to us. Accordingly, we have an obligation to go where people live, but without displacing them or wagging a finger in their faces as to how they should live as we give them love, acceptance, and the care that is the right of all humans. Such care does not seek to supplant cultural roots or lifestyles, but rather to enrich them. The case in point is Haiti and India.

It had been several weeks since I returned from these countries, and thoughts of the damage in Haiti or the poverty in the slums in India kept returning to my mind. I reflected on the purpose, intent, and the meaning of the time I spent in those places. At times, the visions of these communities were blurred. I'd learned from my successes, but I took away much more from my failures—for example, failure to plumb the meaning of what it really means to be less fortunate and allowing people the dignity that family, custom, and place confer on an individual. My experiences in Haiti and India—or anywhere—couldn't be explained in black and white terms. There is discernment involved in knowing what to do and when to do it—and when to leave things the way they are.

When I thought of what we were able to accomplish in Haiti and what we left behind, however, it was hard to sit still and not get going again, back to where life remained dismal and people were already being forgotten because the news cycle had moved on. I realized that we can never use previous experiences as a rationale to feel like we will one day be okay with what we have done, whether in Cambodia, Ethiopia, Kenya, Swaziland, or Egypt. The fact remained that there was much to be done yet in Haiti—and everywhere else, for that matter.

In the end, it all came down to discernment. I knew that, from the largest possible perspective, Medical Mercy was called to aid the less fortunate, and I knew we would continue to visit many countries, including Haiti and India in the near future. But I was humbled by my reflections. As Ecclesiastes says, for everything under heaven there is a time and purpose. There is a time to laugh and weep, plant and sow, dance and mourn, live and die. There is a time to use all of my skills to save a life, and there is a time to discontinue heroic measures for a terminal patient. Every patient, village, country, and trip is different and calls for discernment as to what should be done in a given situation. Yes, people are uniquely different, and only discernment by the grace of His Spirit can inform us what to do for our patients. What I do know is that He, and no one else, decides when it is time to live and when it is time to die.

To everything there is a season, and maybe that reality, as general and incomplete as it may seem, explained my recurring question of why things happen the way they do.

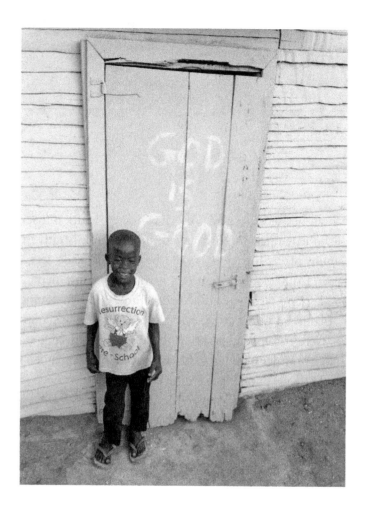

Chapter Twenty
Shantytowns

In March of 2010 we made our third trip to Haiti, our second after the earthquake. With an advanced administrative team already in place so that we would be safe and ready to go, we brought 1,000 pounds of medical supplies, equipment, talking bibles, and tarps with us. Reports indicated that conditions in the country were rough, and simple things like tables and chairs were rudimentary at best. People were suffering a great deal, living under blue tarps, often with no bedding at all, only sheets. When it rained, people got wet and couldn't sleep. Food was scarce, as was almost everything one needed to live even a Spartan existence. The people of Haiti had lived with little, and even that had been taken from them.

Fort National is at the bottom of a hill, a community of about 700 people. The earthquake hit the area hard, and there still hadn't been any significant relief there yet. We found ourselves among many who were sleeping outside, sheltered only by tarps and surrounded by rubble. What we saw was a rebuilding of the community by those who took it upon themselves to do the heavy lifting without any governmental assistance. Within an hour of arriving, we had the clinic up and running, with patients moving from registration to medical examiners, counseling, and the pharmacy. We also gave water purification lessons.

The stories of grief and suffering were numerous and tugged at the heart. Every day, for example, a father wore the shirt his son had on when he died in the earthquake. A grandmother cared for the last of her eight grandchildren, the other seven having died with her daughter, who was the children's mother. A man asked for counseling and prayer because on the night of the earthquake he gave up his bed so that his cousin could sleep inside. He'd slept outside that night, but the building collapsed and his cousin died, leaving the man riddled with guilt. These were stories that one might have expected to read in a stark, depressing novel of literary fiction, but they were all true, and the cast of characters was right by our sides. You'd think we would be depressed with what we were seeing, but mixed in with the tragedy were smiles on the faces of some of the children, as is so often the case.

We went back to Fort National the following morning, holding our clinic in the middle of an area where those who had been displaced slept and lived. They willingly gave up their beds and tables so that we could serve.

I observed a woman for two days. She was alone and had stayed in the same spot every day since the earthquake had struck. She had no friends or family, was mentally handicapped, and withdrawn. No one even knew her name. I talked to the camp leader and asked him to promise that he would personally care for her in exchange for what we were doing for them. We are always quick to run to the children, the ones with the pretty smiles and adorable faces—the ones you want to hug and never let go—but did we do the same for people like her? Or was she too grotesque, too much out of our comfort zone, to hug without letting go or to take a picture with her in order to coax a smile from her expressionless face. I tried but she pulled away. I wanted to try again, but she seemed so far out of reach emotionally that I decided to respect her self-imposed distance. For a day and a half, we walked and worked around her, but I wondered how such a thing could happen—wondered how good a servant I really was. It was situations like this that reminded me of my need to be humble and to feel unashamed around those who are unlike so-called normal people. I would remember her often, hoping she'd felt the touch of my hand if only for a moment.

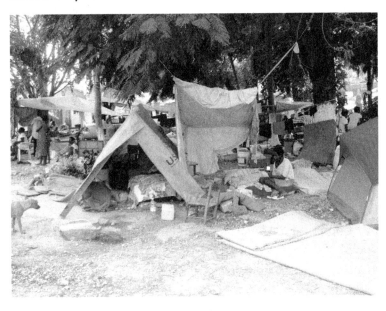

Can you imagine what it would be like if you woke up one morning and found yourself homeless, with no food or water, and your family gone? What if you had no place to go, had nothing, and felt nothing? Dubuisson camp was home for 351 displaced people—about ninety families—who had lost their homes, their loved ones, and had no place to go. They lived in makeshift shelters made of sheets, plastic tarps, gunnysacks, and string. We built shelters, counseled, prayed, taught water filtration, left two water filter systems, and distributed food to the camp. And then we ran out of medicines. We'd seen 890 patients in three days, more than we had expected, with more to come the following day—and the day after that. I wasn't sure what we would do.

Half the team left that morning for Cap-Haitien to check on our One Child Matters children in the projects. About 30,000 refugees had migrated there from Port-au-Prince, and the need was increasing every day for medical help and counseling. Our team primarily did counseling with the children and families in Cap-Haitien while the other half of the team stayed in Port-au-Prince to finish our remaining days of medical clinics, pastoral counseling, and clothing distribution. We returned to Dubuisson camp and saw 130 patients, limiting the number since we were running low on medication and wanted to do some "prayer walking."

All 351 people living in this camp had been displaced from their homes that collapsed during the earthquake. Many were without family members, living in makeshift dwellings constructed from anything they could find in the debris. It was stifling inside these structures, with people sleeping on cinder blocks covered by sheets. They actually tried to cook inside these dwellings, which represented a fire hazard and potential death for the inhabitants. They cooked what little they had, such as the rice and beans we gave them. We'd also brought baby formula powder, clothes, and blankets, which we packaged and distributed to the mothers and the infants they carried, some of them only seventeen days old.

After we finished seeing patients in the afternoon, we broke into pairs and walked the camp with a translator, praying with each of the people living there—our prayer walking. Many tears were shed, many hearts opened, and it was true for us as well as them. I could understand how they'd become almost catatonic in their emotions—tearless and empty. At the end of the day, however, there was the slightest hint of a smile on the faces of some, a look of hope and a genuine expression of thanks from some of the Haitians. They thought they had been forgotten, but we proved that to be false. God knew who they were and what they had suffered, and as usual, we were only His instruments.

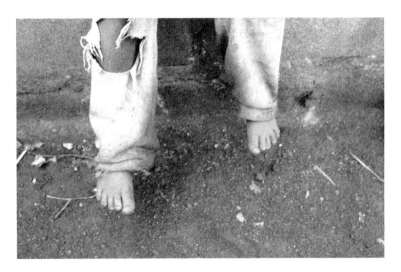

It rained the fourth night we were there. We thought of those in Dubuisson and how wet and miserable they must be in their makeshift dwellings, with even their sheets getting wet.

We decided to go back to Dubuisson, but on the fifth day we went to Ave Fouchard, a city-based community. Although devastated, it seemed to be moving in the direction of recovery. Upon arrival, we found ourselves in an empty lot at the end of a one-way path, with one way in and one way out. A steel gate separated us from the crowd that grew outside, waiting for our services.

We saw patients in a makeshift clinic and then left for God's Little Angels orphanage, which we learned of when we were in Haiti immediately following the earthquake. A small newborn, Baby Jude, was brought to us by his mother, who asked us to care for him. He was severely dehydrated and in dire straits. We put in an IV, resuscitated him, and gave him to the orphanage, where he thrived for a short time, growing and actually becoming chunky. He subsequently developed an intestinal infection and lost weight, so we put Baby Jude back on IV fluids and meds, and he started to recover again. I just recently learned that he thrived and is now a young boy growing and doing well.

It wasn't getting any easier each day as we treated the seemingly endless cases lined up at our registration tables. The team in Cap-Haitien had a particularly rough day. They counseled over a hundred people, many of them children, but almost all of them related stories of pain and grief. We'd heard the same in Port-au-Prince. Stories of loss were everywhere. All anyone really needs is God's love and grace, but it's hard for people who have lost everything to live from a place of deep spirituality, and although we counseled and prayed with them, we remained nonjudgmental and accepted their mindset and blank stares. We knew that many did not feel God's presence and love, but it was surely there. There are those who voluntarily strip themselves of worldly possessions in order to become religious hermits or monks, but poverty had been forced on an already-decimated population because of the earthquake. And yet they came to us, and that expressed hope, and where there is hope He always is at our sides, walking with us to Emmaus even when we don't recognize Him.

Even Jesus knew what it was like not to have a home since His full humanity coexisted with His divinity. He said that "Birds of the air have nests, and foxes have holes, but the Son of Man has nowhere to lay his head." Such was the case for the homeless and sick in Haiti, living in shanties made of tarps, plywood, corrugated tin, and anything they could find. These dwellings weren't real homes, and the people had no place to lay their heads except on earth, wood, or concrete. God Himself had lived that way, and I was sure that His love was in their hearts even if they didn't feel it.

Our last day in Haiti was one of both fun and sadness. We finished up in the camp where need was the greatest. After six days in Port-au-Prince, we'd seen 1,300 patients, pastored and counseled over 500 people, built shelters, delivered water filtration systems, fed 300 people for a week, taught basic hygiene to children, had a question and answer session with mothers about taking care of their babies, danced and sang with the community, and witnessed a strengthened faith in many of those we'd treated. Before we'd landed, we had no preconceived notion of how it would all turn out, and no pretense of thinking that we were going to make a significant difference in what had happened to Haiti. Had we?

Jesus taught a beautiful parable that says the following: "This is what the kingdom of God is like. A man throws seed on the land. Night and day, while he sleeps, when he is awake, the seed is sprouting and growing; how he does not know. Of its own accord "the land produces first the shoot, then the ear, then the full grain in the ear" (Mark 4: 26-28). We can't always know how or when things will happen, but they do according to a plan beyond our meetings and emails and charter flights. They happen of their "own accord."

During a team meeting, a question was asked on our last night: were we giving enough? The answer turned out to be relatively simple. It depended on the definition of giving. Materially and medically, we couldn't because of the scope of the disaster. The same held true for providing food and shelter. But what we were able to give was everlasting and never ending, love and care that would be passed on to others. It's called agape, or the unconditional, selfless love of one person for another.

We weren't quite sure what would happen in Haiti, but with agape love we made a difference. Haiti is a small country, but it's a part of His kingdom. Seed was planted there and grew by its own accord. Even now, years later, I trust that a crop is still growing, one that is lovingly looked after by the One who guides all things.

Chapter Twenty-one
Slum Dogs and Mustard Seeds

After twenty-four hours of flying, we arrived in New Delhi in May of 2010 to start five days of clinics in three poverty-stricken slums. We would be treating patients, primarily children, in the projects centered in these slums. We checked into the hotel, showered, and then met in a conference room to package and label over 10,000 doses of medicine. That equaled 10,000 prescriptions projected over a five-day period, but as happens on most trips, we knew we'd run out of meds and have to replenish our supplies. As we move into the week on a typical mission, more and more people hear that we're in their region, and the clinics swell. We can never predict just how much medicine we'll need, but the most important thing we bring never runs out, which is grace and compassion. Holding a hand, praying, hugging, laughing, and telling those who come to see us that we care about them is sometimes all the medicine they need.

We began our five days of clinics with an unexpected treat. Before we even started on the first day, we had garlands placed around our necks by the children, gifts freely given and humbly received. We were at The Life Center Academy, which was a Christian-run school located in New Delhi's Satya Nikethan district, an urban area surrounded by slums. Twenty-five percent of the population in the slums fell below the poverty line, and of these, over forty percent of the children had no access to any kind of education. The Life Center Academy's primary aim was to cater to these children and provide them with an education that they wouldn't receive under normal circumstances. The academy also had a school for children with special needs, such as mental retardation, hearing disabilities, speech disorders, autism, and others. The hope was that they could one day be integrated into the main school.

We worked nonstop, breaking for forty-five minutes to grab a Chinese lunch before resuming work. For the most part, the children were relatively healthy, but malnutrition affected almost forty percent of them. We did a comprehensive nutritional assessment on children using a computer program that calculated their nutritional status. We learned that visual impressions were not necessarily to be trusted. The healthiest child often turned out to be moderately malnourished. With such a fact so easily missed, children were at risk for delayed development and possibly early death. As a result of the assessment, I put together a comprehensive nutritional rescue program that would hopefully make a difference in the children's lives within six months of their participation in it.

Abandoned children were found, rescued, and cared for, and some even seemed happy, but the sad cases were present as always. An eleven-year-old girl was found in a part of the city known for prostitution and brought to One Child Matters. She complained of abdominal pain, after which I took her aside and, with a female interpreter, gently asked her questions that could help me determine whether or not she had been sexually harmed and if she had a sexually transmitted disease. She tearfully shared her story—she had indeed suffered abuse—but she was treated, counseled, and loved, as she always should have been. She accepted our care, and a precious life was given a new path, one offering hope and dignity.

After a forty-five-minute drive, we came to a main street packed with tuk-tuks (three-wheel automotive taxis), over-crowded buses, people carrying a variety of goods on their heads, cows, and bicycles loaded with merchandise, each of which had a command of the traffic and ruled the right of way. It was India, where cattle are sacred and people are dispensable. Across the main street was Kalkaji, the slum that was to be our place of work for the day.

We saw 400 children, and malnutrition was rampant. Over seventy percent of the children we treated were grossly under-weight and moderately or severely malnourished. We saw two twelve-year-old children who weighed thirty-five and forty-four pounds respectively. One of these children was named Rocky—his real name—and he captured our hearts. Rocky was twelve and weighed thirty-five pounds and was forty-four inches tall.

As we packed up, a ten-year-old boy was brought in seizing, We quickly went into resuscitation mode but unfortunately didn't have the right drugs to stop the seizures. We gave him fluids, IV antibiotics, and sent him to the hospital.

The truth is that all of the children capture our hearts, which is why it's so agonizing when we can't do more to help each and every one.

Once in a while we realize that all things are possible, es-pecially when we believe they are, and the following day bore that out. A gifted U.S. Medical Mercy team, working with an incredible Indian team from a One Child Matters project, saw 600 patients in one day. It happened without fanfare, with medical examinations performed, prescriptions handed out, patients prayed with, and with not one complaint, excuse, or question. Through it all, I saw silent servants giving of themselves for others. Jesus said that if we had faith the size of a mustard seed, we could move mountains and that all things would be possible. I believe that when we're at our best, praying and believing, mountains are moved. It's not always so easy to retain that mindset when dealing with some of our more difficult cases, but we renew ourselves daily with prayer. Do miracles happen? I firmly believe they do.

We returned to the same slum community where we'd been the day before. As I mentioned earlier, there are over 2,000 children who are cared for by the ministry of Pastor Koshy and his wife Joicy. Six hundred of those are One Child Matters children. We decided to see as many as possible, and we managed to treat 1,000 of the children, and that, too, was miraculous in its own way. We are told in the Gospel that five loaves of bread fed five thousand people. Sometimes, our time is multiplied as well. At the end of a long day, we sometimes realize that we've seen far more patients than is reasonably possible. We don't question the numbers, however. We give thanks and move on.

The slum community was rife with evil. Parents sold their children for $500 to gangs, never to be seen again, just to feed their drug habit. Girls as young as twelve were married off and had children by the age of thirteen. I examined a twenty-six-year-old woman who already had five children, giving birth to her first in her early teens. Her husband was a drug addict, abused her, and sold her on a regular basis. Pastor Koshy and I spent a lot of time with her since one of her children was a sponsored child of One Child Matters. Wringing her hands, she never looked at us or shed a tear as she told her story. It was obvious that she'd lost her emotions. As always, there was no judgment on our part. Who is to say what people might do—even ourselves—when faced with the horrors of the slum? We examined Hindu and Muslim children who applied dark makeup to their eyes to ward off evil spirits. We looked past the things we didn't understand or agree with and took care of those who came to us. Judgment is for someone greater than us.

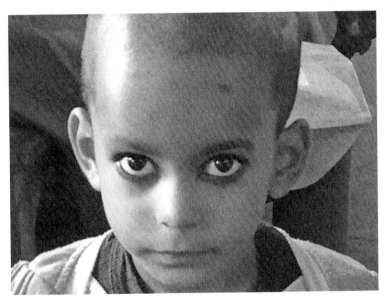

The slum, a place called home by many lost souls, was beyond description. The cramped feeling—the extreme closeness of living with nine other people in a small room four feet by eight feet—can only be understood by standing in it as I did. I felt the darkness bury my senses until I finally had to escape and come up for air, so to speak. The inhabitants, however, knew no other life. It all comes back to understanding that such people have a strong sense of place, of home, regardless of how wretched their conditions may be. By the same token, that never prohibits us from praying that God will lead the inhabitants of slums to places of light, health, and freedom.

Given such conditions, is it really true that all things are possible? Six of the teachers that worked in this slum—and who worked with us that day—were once themselves "slum dogs." They were taken in by Pastor Koshy and Joicy at the age of twelve and were sponsored by those who cared enough to love from a distance. They all "graduated" from this project, went on to get their teaching degrees, and came back to the place they had escaped from. One day, maybe the little girl who was saved from being sold to the gangs will also become a teacher, caring for those who are forgotten.

We are told to pray to the Lord of the harvest, that He might send laborers into his field, where the harvest is rich. We see fields ripe with potential miracles everywhere we go. If six can do it, then others can as well, but perhaps the miracles start with one trip at a time—and one person at a time finding health, grace, and an inner joy that was previously absent. Mustard seed faith doesn't look like much at the beginning, but it can grow and blossom into new lives, into miracles.

As you might recall, Sangam Vihar—the Rag Picker slum—was the place where garbage was currency, and children sorted through toxic dumps to find plastic for wealthy owners and their middlemen. Here, too, young girls were sold to the sex trade, and people were kidnapped, drugged, and operated on, only to wake up and find that both of their kidneys had been removed and sold for a great deal of money. In turn, they, too, died unless they could find the money to pay for someone else's kidneys. Seeing life in the Rag Picker slum close up was a challenge to my thoughts on miracles, of people escaping a toxic life that was the result of living in toxic conditions, both literally and figuratively. Did such places signal that there was a limit to what God could do? Was I to adopt more realistic expectations?

These questions came as they usually do, but the exhortation to faith remains. After Jesus cursed a fig tree that bore no fruit, the tree withered immediately, astonishing His followers. Jesus' response was very straightforward: "I tell you therefore: everything you ask and pray for, believe that you have it already, and it will be yours" (Mark 11:24/JB)). It's interesting to note that this verse of scripture hinges on the future tense. It *will* be yours. With darkness, corruption, and evil in Sangam Vihar being so extensive—even palpable—it was hard to believe that change would come, but the Letter to the Hebrews in the New Testament tells us that faith is the "assurance of things not hoped for, the conviction of things not seen." Again, the emphasis is on the future, and that is the heart of faith: expectation when expectation is neither reasonable nor logical. I could only trust that His light could penetrate even the darkest heart, the darkest situation. I realized that I couldn't look at only the present moment, but the promise and hope that all situations contain in seed form, a promise of redemption.

A seed is only a seed when it's planted. It's destiny, however, is to grow into something entirely different and to break through the darkness of the soil where it begins its life. And perhaps that is the deeper sadness of the third world: people have written it off. They expect nothing good to come from it, but I've been there and know better. His hand is moving. He's there, and seeds are growing.

We finished our last day of medical clinics, and in five days saw 2,000 patients, dispensed over 10,000 prescriptions, and prayed more than one would think humanly possible. The remorse of not being able to do more was offset by the sense of hope that I found there. When I looked back at the days we spent working in some of the worst slums in the world, I saw specks of light in the otherwise dark cloud hanging over the lives of those people. There were the smiles of children, tearful expressions of thanks from parents, and the soft touch of a calloused hand that had felt nothing but garbage its entire life. These gave me solace because those we served had experienced the warmth of dignity, the pride of being recognized as human, and a love they hadn't felt for a very long time. While saddened by the indignities they suffered, I knew we had to let go of the rational thoughts trying to sabotage our minds with hopelessness. It would be easy to harbor the mental images we had from our days in the slums of India, but those pictures needed to be burned. We knew firsthand what it was like to be a slum dog, but it was the rays of light that were angling into the dark recesses of the slums that counted, light that came to heal those whose lives were regarded as so much garbage. It was the seed under the soil, under the garbage, that counted.

The Book of Revelation tells us that one day the entire earth will be transformed and redeemed. It won't happen overnight, but that's the way of seeds. You plant them, step back, and then water them with hope. It's what we've been commanded to do.

Chapter Twenty-two

Loaves and Fishes

In August of 2010 I heard the news that medical missionaries were killed in Afghanistan because of their evangelization efforts. The team members of Medical Mercy have found ourselves on some occasions falling within the boundaries of such hatred and danger. Thankfully, we have been protected by common sense, trust, security details, evacuation protocols, and code words. Most of all we have been protected by faith. But hadn't the medical missionaries who were murdered also relied on faith? If so, how was it different for us? It wasn't, really. We open ourselves up to danger with each trip, praying that it won't happen and thankful for when it doesn't. Even with precautions, however, anything can happen. I am always mindful that we frequently treat patients in areas surrounded by gangs, drugs, and sex trafficking, but that is where the need is and that is where we are told to go. St. Paul's ministry to the very first Christian communities was not without peril, and neither is ours, but like him, we trust the Spirit is always with us. With these thoughts in mind, I and my team were ready to depart for Kenya on August 20th, for I was also aware that somewhere there were children who hadn't had a good night's sleep in a long time because they were hungry, sick, alone, or scared.

We made it to Malindi via Nairobi. About one and a half hours out of Malindi—using all dirt roads to get there—we set up a clinic, examined patients under a tent, and dispensed medicine from a mud building. It was radically different from my routine in the States, where a few days earlier I'd taken care of severely ill and injured children in a ten-million-dollar pediatric intensive care unit—and with everything I needed. In Kenya, it was dirt, sand, mud huts, mosquitoes, medicine out of boxes and baggies, a generator to power a computer used for nutritional assessment data, no bathrooms, and children who had never seen a doctor. Not surprisingly, the life expectancy was only thirty-five years. Was one place better than the other?

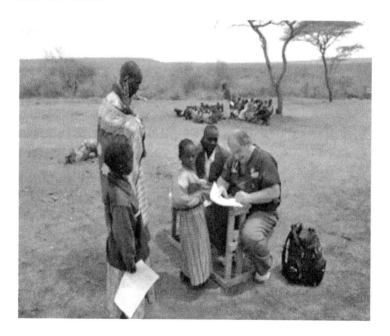

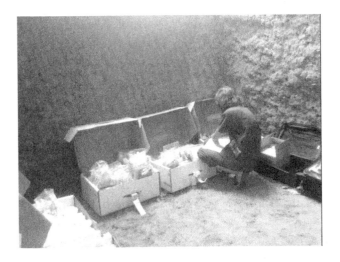

The technology and the availability of medical supplies in the United States, or course, trumped what we had in Kenya, but that didn't represent the entire picture. In Kenya and the other countries we visited, there were acts of giving with no expectation of what would be received in return. There were no insurance forms, no billing, no co-pays, just agape—that unconditional love. In short, we had covenant relationships. I saw it in the healthcare workers the first time they held the hand of a patient who had come to them for help. They took those hands and held tightly, unafraid, gracious, and caring. Unfortunately, such care is lacking in some of the largest hospitals in the United States and other developed countries.

On some days things just don't seem fair, and day two of our trip was one of those days. We saw over 200 patients in a village with mud huts and a lot of vegetation. The weather varied between light rain and bursts of sunshine throughout the day. We saw malnutrition and a host of other diseases, and we all agreed that the children we treated were sicker than those from the day before. There was also a clear difference between the health of the children who were sponsored and those who were not. The sponsored children were sick, but the others were much sicker, which affirmed that One Child Matters gives children a far better chance at life. But what of those who were *not* sponsored? We saw two children who had significant medical problems that could have been addressed, but due to their non-sponsored status, they were not going to be helped since they had complex medical issues that would have involved a great deal of resources, time, and commitment—unless we decided to intervene. The sadness of it all was that if they had received the kind of treatment that sponsored children did, both would have been able to live longer and better lives.

We struggled with the question of whether we should jump in and start the process of diagnostic tests, referrals to specialists, and recommending advanced medical care as opposed to leaving well enough alone. Unless we were committed to seeing it all the way through, which would entail years of specialized medical care, we would only give these children false hope for a better future. To start a process and then abandon it halfway through just didn't make sense. Regrettably, we decided that the right thing to do was not to start a process that couldn't be finished. It sounded cold, but without full commitment, the children living in the bush of Kenya would have become more disillusioned with life than they were before as they waited for a cure that would never come. There is nothing worse than a broken heart resulting from a broken promise, but this is the reality of third world medicine. There are some things we just can't do. We turn away often, hoping that those we can't help don't see the tears in our eyes.

Life isn't fair. We helped a lot of children but walked away from two who needed more than we could give. It was yet another case in which God would watch two small sparrows fall from the sky. I could only give them to Him and trust in His larger purposes.

The next day went smoothly and lifted my spirits. We conducted the clinic outside, with the wind blowing and the tarps flapping. We were gifted with traditional Kenyan ware and with love from the children. Things went so well, in fact, that I found myself asking disturbing questions when I lay down that night, questions that again revolved around the issue of contrasts.

Sleep can wax and wane, receding into wakefulness for hours. In my case, it may have been due to jet lag or just a desire to find answers. We were in Kenya after months of planning, the date having been set a year earlier following a lot of coordination, emailing, purchasing, and organizing, but my thoughts suddenly turned to my life back home. We'd done a great job in Kenya and the other places we'd gone, helping the forgotten children to the extent that we were able to do so. With prayer, we always center ourselves on what is important, and that means focusing on others. But when we go back to the U.S., we have families, friends, jobs, activities, hobbies, and everything that makes us happy. That was the phrase that caused me to reflect: "Makes us happy." What would it be like if we went back home with the same mindset that we had in Kenya, one of obedience, giving, charity, kindness, love, and grace? What if that attitude was never ending and always present? Being in Kenya brought out the best in us. It felt nice and warm, heart filling and rewarding. We felt loved and gave that love back as we cared for the less fortunate. Was I like that all the time in the United States? Probably not. That's what kept me awake—trying to understand how easy it was to be wonderfully giving to the children and families we saw in the countries we traveled to, and how hard it was to do the same back home. Sometimes, I concluded, I wasn't a good steward of my gifts.

The gospel tells us that Jesus could work no miracles when he returned to his home town of Nazareth. To the people there, Jesus was someone they'd seen grow up. He was just another face, not a savior or miracle worker, and yet He was the Son of God. It's easy to look beyond the extraordinary—to miss seeing Him—when one assumes the daily routines of life. I realized, however, that it wasn't realistic to always live one's "peak experience" or constantly exist on a spiritual plateau. The Gospel even tells us that Jesus Himself grew tired, hungry, and thirsty at times—even frustrated when His disciples failed to grasp His teaching. It's part of being human. The good news is that I also realized that I was a little better because of the trips, able to retain love, humility, and faith even when not ministering in slums and clinics around the world.

I fell asleep, content to know that God understood who I and my team were. Our hearts were aimed in the right direction.

I'd come to Kenya exactly one year earlier to give a one-week course for pastors and teachers who worked with us during our week of clinics. It was a program designed to help healthcare workers recognize a sick child, start basic treatment, and know when to transfer him or her to an advanced healthcare facility. This week represented the second phase of their training—their practical, or skills training—when they actually saw patients with us and put into practice what they'd learned in class. The training was intense, and the learning curve steep. By the end of the week, healthcare workers were seeing patients on their own. They also learned how to dispense medications and do nutritional assessments.

We had a graduation dinner and ceremony for these selfless workers and handed out their certificates, with each receiving a bag filled with medical supplies and medicines that they would use in the projects. It was a wonderful end to a wonderful week. Pastor Daniel, who was both a pastor and one of our healthcare workers, shared that he'd saved a woman's life a few months earlier because he had learned the Heimlich maneuver. In turn, he had taught it to his community members, and two of them had used it on family members who'd been choking on food. Pastor Daniel also said that many of the parents of the children seen were touched by the fact that their own people, their community of pastors and teachers, had given of themselves to help others in unexpected ways. The patients and parents were comforted by the fact that the hands that touched them were familiar hands and part of their culture. Finally, Pastor Daniel said that he'd learned that the most powerful medicine they brought to patients was the gift of themselves. This was tremendous validation that the good we bring to a country extends far beyond five to seven days of treating patients. Through grace, God multiplies the initial care we bring—the loaves and fishes, if you will—so that many more can be helped long after a Medical Mercy team has left. A technique as simple yet important as the Heimlich maneuver had saved lives. Love and concern were already spreading simply because workers native to the region were using our hands-on techniques. Prayer, medical care, hope, love—it was all continuing thanks to a power that can do infinitely more than we can possibly ask for or imagine (Ephesians 3: 20).

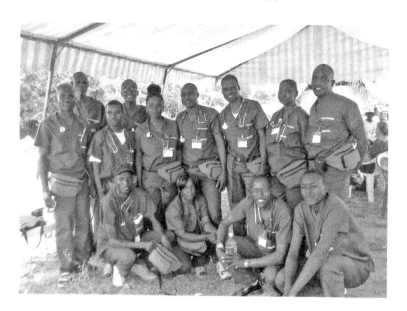

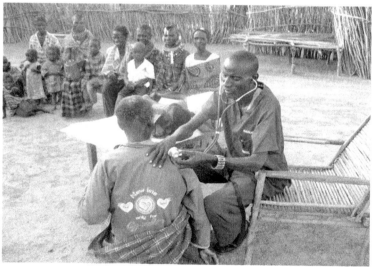

This is what brings us back to countries like Kenya. Despite all our shortcomings, which are many, we found light and guidance in the words of people such as Pastor Daniel, who had reassured us that what we do makes a difference. He also gave me even greater humility. While I may not always live up to my own expectations, I understood that, as St. Paul puts it, God is greatest when we are weak. He makes up for our shortcomings and turns everything to the good. I understood that even manpower, such as the healthcare workers, multiplied when I was back in Phoenix with my eye not constantly focused on a clinic in the slum or the bush. The workers, in turn, kept multiplying the skills and love we had instilled in them. As the saying goes, not bad work when you can get it.

The interesting thing about the story of Jesus multiplying the loaves and fishes, a story that is described in all four gospels, is that not only did five loaves and two fish feed over five thousand people, but when the meal was finished, the disciples collected a dozen basketfuls of leftovers that could be used to feed even more people. Nothing was wasted, although this last part of the story is often overlooked.

It was this aspect of God's abundance that impressed me. I'd come up against unfairness in the form of two unsponsored children who wouldn't get the long-term care they needed. But who is to say that somewhere down the line at a time when we are safely back in our American homes that these children would not find a miracle? Who is to say that in the baskets of God's overflowing goodness, there will not be a little left over for those in need? I may never see it happen personally, but Jesus assures us that justice comes even when it is delayed. This is not to say that everyone finds everything they need in third world countries. Obviously they don't. But with people like Pastor Daniel, I believe that some people do find miracles. Why? Because I've seen them multiply firsthand.

Chapter Twenty-three
Cholera in Haiti

A team was leaving for Cambodia in November of 2010, but I wasn't going to be with them. Ten months after the earthquake in Haiti, a severe cholera epidemic hit the island, and I made an assessment trip to see just how bad things were and what would be needed there. I learned that cholera was present in Cap-Haitien and Lembe and that One Child Matters was gathering data on the living conditions of registered children. It was also trying to identify which water filtration systems were being used and which ones weren't.

Several of our children were critically ill, and some had already died. Parents, church members, and pastors were all affected. Our general plan was to bring some semblance of health care and prevention to those who were suffering. There was civil unrest and riots, and the question of our safety would be a real concern.

Complicating issues was the fact that a presidential election had recently been held in Haiti. There had been nineteen candidates, fifteen of which claimed there had been fraud at the ballot box. With an announcement of the winner expected within twenty-four to forty-eight hours, demonstrations and violence were expected. Meanwhile, I was in the States, assessing what cholera was doing to our children in the projects.

Haiti seemed to exist in a state of perpetual hardship. In the midst of crippling poverty, there had been first an earthquake and then a cholera epidemic. It has been said that a mouse will kick an elephant when it's down. A large mouse was kicking, and the country was going to be down for quite a while.

Within fifteen minutes of landing in Cap-Haitien, I visited Justinian Hospital and a cholera treatment center (CTC). Within two hours, we established the referral pattern for our sickest children and collaborated with the Baptist Hospital in Carrefour La Mort, where a cholera treatment center was being set up. I decided to visit these facilities before heading to the projects since I would need a place to refer the sicker children I would encounter. People were coming by the hundreds, and I made quick rounds and saw row upon row of dehydrated and sick patients receiving treatment. A triage system was set up based on A) oral rehydration, B) oral/IV rehydration and observation, and C) treating seriously ill and dying patients. Chlorine basins were everywhere since chlorine effectively kills several pathogens, such as typhoid, dysentery, cholera, and others. Even our shoes were sprayed with chlorine when we left the area.

Thanks to Jack from the One Child Matters headquarters, and the country coordinator for the program, many basic steps had already been taken in the projects. Each project had two people designated as "prevention specialists," who'd been trained by us to teach hand washing, waste disposal, assessment of dehydration, and general hygiene. Each family had received a gallon of chlorine for their water, a new water filter, five one-pound blocks of soap, and packets of oral rehydration solution. Thus far, everything seemed to be working, a huge first step in stopping the spread of the disease. Additionally, assessments were planned for latrines, sewage, and waste disposal.

It had been a long day. I hoped the following day would bring calm, with no civil unrest to compromise our efforts. There was so much to do, and I felt like precious time and lives were slipping away. When I closed my eyes, I saw the humiliation of people lying in their own diarrhea, people who were dehydrated and dying. I could only imagine what they themselves saw when they closed their eyes. Did the infected people of Haiti have any hope left, or were they too sick?

When you think everything is under control and going smoothly, something can grab your attention and take over very quickly. An eight-year-old boy did that on my second day. We went to three projects to look at a group of children who were identified the previous week as needing a more thorough look-see. Jack and Edrice had done a competent preliminary assessment of the children and identified those who looked moderately or severely ill and dehydrated. It was now my turn to examine them. I saw one hundred children from the three projects, referred fourteen of them for further care, and had one child transported to a cholera treatment center. He was the one who got my attention. He was eight but looked five. He was severely dehydrated and malnourished, more than likely from being ill for a while. He was lethargic, pale, and had a weak pulse. Frankly, I thought he would collapse in a matter of hours. We rushed him to the CTC, and he was immediately treated after I consulted with the physician there. By the time we left, he was getting IV therapy and was on a comprehensive fluid resuscitation protocol that the local physician and I put together. We also planned a one-week nutritional rescue program for him that would ensure his recovery. Without Jack's and others preliminary exam of the boy, I have no doubt that he would have died.

We established a relationship with two hospitals that would take our children and care for them when needed, this being essential so that the sicker children wouldn't slip through the cracks or lack for want of a higher level of care. We met with several physicians and discussed long-term plans for cholera prevention and intervention. Cholera was in Haiti to stay for a while, but our projects were ahead of the game by having chlorine, soap, and education in place.

I was very encouraged with what I'd seen and with what we had been able to do for our children, but as I moved through the country, there was still evidence of the toll that cholera was taking. I came across a young woman sitting in a wheel chair, an IV in her arm and a blank stare on her face. Rice water stool dripped from her wheel chair, but she was unaware of the pool of diarrhea that was accumulating beneath her. People walked around her, staring. I stopped briefly to touch her arm and tell her that I was not ashamed to be next to her, to let her know that she, too, should not be ashamed. I turned and left, knowing that she might not make it. I could only hope that she felt my touch and knew that I was not afraid of her or her illness. Cholera in Haiti carries a stigma no different than AIDS did many years ago, with people reticent to be near those affected. She deserved more than the stares and fear of people who circled her chair, as if she were quarantined or on display in a museum of the dying. She'd become a what—someone infected—not a who.

As bad as things were, we were making a difference. Every life saved—every patient practicing preventative measures—meant that the disease had less of a chance to spread farther into the population. I took a deep breath and moved on, planning to travel to more projects the following day.

⌒⌒

I was at the border of Haiti and the Dominican Republic on my third day. Cholera can unfortunately travel quickly and without discrimination. We visited four of our projects, and I examined over 100 children and found them all to be healthy. A few had chronic illnesses, but at least there were no signs of cholera in our children. The prophylactic measures were making a bigger difference than I thought even though the projects were in very remote places, with filth everywhere.

I saw a little child sitting on his mother's bed. The woman was critically ill with cholera—it was written on her face. I couldn't walk away without making sure that this fragile woman was going to make it. I spoke with the medical team caring for her and went over their plans, suggesting a slight change in therapy, and we all agreed she would pull through. I couldn't accept anything less.

Jesus healed large crowds, but he did so one person at a time, and occasionally His attention was directed to a single individual by those desperate for a healing, either for themselves or a relative. He didn't stand on a large hill and simply zap everyone with His power. Everyone received personal attention; everyone received a touch from the savior's hand. If we act in His name, we can do no less. As the name implies, one child matters—and so do adults, such as the woman in the wheelchair or the mother on the bed.

Day four was good, at least for the children in our projects in Quanamenthe. We saw children from seven projects and the orphanage, and I examined about 150 who looked sick. Thankfully, only a few needed referrals to a clinic, and none needed urgent attention. All in all, cholera had met its match, at least in our own projects. Chlorine was being used, soap was being lathered up, and the children were happy. I visited the local hospital and spoke to the organization that was setting up another cholera treatment center, pleased with what was available for our children if needed. Additionally, sixty-five of our project representatives were becoming prevention specialists, responsible for continuous cholera prevention and education. Sometimes the road to progress is less cluttered than expected, and for that I was thankful. On the other side of the wall, however—outside of our projects—there was still much devastation. Our children were the lucky ones.

The questions asked by those training to be prevention specialists were interesting: if cholera was in the water and the fish, was it safe to swim in the ocean?; why were the dead burned and not buried?; where did cholera start?; could you get cholera more than once?; and what did cholera look like? I spoke on the cause of cholera and its prevention, assessment, and treatment. We ended the week with a powerful take-home message: no one should die of cholera, and no one should get it. Hygiene and sanitation were the keys to prevention, and fluid, fluid, fluid was the mainstay of therapy. Hydration was crucial.

I don't think it's an accident that water is such a powerful symbol in almost all world religions, especially Christianity. It is a sign of cleansing, as seen in baptism, of washing away that which corrupts and destroys. In the Gospel of John, Jesus cried out that streams of living water would flow from anyone who believed in Him. And when passing through Samaria, Jesus sat down at a well and asked a woman for a drink of water, telling her that He Himself had a different kind of water, water that would never leave her thirsty again.

It's also a fact that sixty percent of our bodies is made of water, which is why hydration is so important when treating almost any illness. There is therefore spiritual water—grace, if you will—and literal water. Both cleanse, both sustain, and both heal. The water filtration systems we distribute filter out the dirt, making it potable. The prayers we say with our patients hopefully confer grace and faith, filtering out different kinds of impurities, those that taint the spirit.

Nothing good comes from cholera, of course, but every situation is an opportunity to learn, a reminder of what's real and important. The necessity for clean water in Haiti following the cholera outbreak was a reminder both medical and spiritual. Good covenant care, as we've seen, is holistic. Whether we confer in His name pure drinking water or the waters of grace, we are caring for body and spirit. But it all starts with prayer. With the right supplies, we can heal the body, but the soul is the real source of life. And if our patients aren't Christian—if they're Hindu, Muslim, or Buddhist—that's fine, too. We pray with them as well if they allow us to do so, for everyone's soul needs God's grace, God's cleansing.

Water. Grace. The words themselves are beautiful when pronounced. God can heal so many things, whether it's cholera, malnutrition, abuse, neglect, garbage, filth, or unfairness. He can heal in the city, project, or bush. Most importantly, He can heal and renew our minds. And so I wonder: whether we heal the body or the spirit, are we not having an impact on the other, directly or indirectly? I suspect that, as a result of the Creator's wisdom, healing flows in both directions. It's what covenant medicine is all about.

Chapter Twenty-four
Sustainability

It's odd to get a glimpse of something you know well from a time somewhere in the distant past. I'd seen cholera when I was the director of pediatrics in the Cambodian refugee camp thirty-two years earlier. In fact, there had been two epidemics: measles and cholera, and I contracted measles encephalitis and was evacuated to a Bangkok ICU for a week. Back at the camp, I learned about cholera quickly and how to treat it. I hadn't had to use that knowledge again until a few months earlier, when Haiti brought back all those memories. The memory of my time in Cambodia offered a valuable reminder that things sometimes don't change, such as poor sanitation, bad hygiene, and dirty water. I was a little heavier now, and yes a lot heavier and with a lot less hair, but much wiser from my experiences when thirty, and so it was back to Haiti yet again.

With considerable effort, the twin engine thirty-seat passenger plane lifted off the runway in Fort Lauderdale, fully loaded and short on fuel. One sacrifices fuel for passengers and baggage—that's the law of lift and weight in an airplane. We landed an hour later on a small island in the Bahamas to refuel and make our way to Cap-Haitien. Three hours after that we were at our first clinic, where we did physicals, nutritional assessments, identified those who were malnourished, conducted cholera education, and distributed vitamins. We saw a community of children who positively loved being loved.

The filth was still present, of course. Stagnant water, algae, and garbage surrounded the children. They lived, played, and slept in it, and it was hard to imagine how they made it from day to day. But because of our aggressive cholera education and prevention program on our four previous trips, we saw only a handful of children who had cholera—all of them were doing well—with no new cases presenting. Our quick response and initiative when the epidemic started had paid off.

And what a difference food makes. A few calories, a little protein, carbohydrates, and unsaturated fats can give a child an opportunity to grow and live, and that's what we saw: well-fed children, which was a testimony to the protocol of feeding children in the projects at least once a week, if not more. This is not to say that we didn't see any children who were malnourished, because we did, but their number was in the minority. When nutritional supplement was called for, we used Medika Mamba, a paste made from ground peanuts, powdered milk, sugar, oil, and vitamins.

We came, treated, prayed, and loved, which is the short but accurate description of what our goal is for every trip we make. We ran three parallel tracts: physical exams, cholera education, and nutritional assessment and rescue. I hoped that the children who we saw today would one day do the same for others, and I was confident that many would. We'd seen many individuals in the countries we visited pay it forward to their brothers and sisters in need—and to God.

You would think that there would always be something dramatic to write about given the nature of my work—some amazing miracle story or the tale of a child who stood out because of some special need. The truth is, that's not always the case. Except for one child, our second day in Haiti was one of those days. We went to three projects and saw a total of 180 children. There was no drama, just beautiful children and a whole lot of love. And that was the point, wasn't it—180 healthy children, all smiling and playing? It meant that Medical Mercy was working for these children in all of its stated goals.

As for the one child that caught our attention, Dr. Dave (a physician who assisted on the trip) saw the child of a worker in the project. This young child had cerebral palsy and was already showing signs of significant arm and leg stiffness. With genuine compassion and encouragement, he explained to the mother why the child was like this. God's love for all, regardless of who or what they are was his message. He also told her how blessed the child was to have a loving mother like herself. It struck me that his words were the words that our God continually speaks to us: He loves us unconditionally with compassion and grace. When I reflected on how the children were doing, I realized anew that our success was due to this unconditional love, which can never be exhausted or minimized. Whenever Jesus met with sinners, the sick, and the contrite, he spoke with compassion and love, and Dr. Dave had done exactly that.

The next day wasn't so easy, however. We went to two projects, both in the direction of the border with the Dominican Republic. We saw many children with chronic illnesses, which I thought we'd had under control. There was a new wave of illnesses that had cropped up and we attacked them: skin infections, pneumonia, pustules, and many more. Had we missed something a year ago? No, illness occurs in some places more than others, and that's why we traveled to Haiti and other countries again and again: to make sure we were doing what needed to be done. We dealt with the diseases and gave the children a chance to live a better life. We can't ever guarantee a successful outcome for any given patient, but if we give them a chance at a healthy future and demonstrate the virtues of love as we counsel and pray with them, then we've done our job. Even in a healthy population, an individual with hope will almost always do better in all aspects of life than someone who feels defeated. We left these children with good care, medicine, follow-up protocols, and a great deal of hope, and that brings smiles to our own faces as well every single time.

Most of the team remained in Haiti, seeing children in five additional clinics and working at the orphanage, washing clothes, doing construction, and caring for the forty-six children that we had there. I returned to Phoenix to give scheduled lectures at the medical school, where I taught the Ethics and Medical Humanism curriculum. But we'd accomplished what we went there to do: provide cholera education, nutritional assessment and rescue, and physical exams. It was interesting that we went with the expectation that conditions had probably deteriorated due to cholera, but we returned with the satisfaction that all the preparation, intervention, and educational programs had worked. It had been a case on my part of favoring caution over confidence, but since we'd avoided getting self-righteous about who we were and what we did, things had turned out well. As I mentioned above, it's not about guarantees, but about giving chances, and that's a goal that calls for humility, for we always place matters, long-term and short, in God's hands. What was striking was the humility that each team member had demonstrated, for too many times I've seen concern glazed over by superiority complexes. Our team, however, was solid, and I was proud of their hard work and dedication. It was, and still is, always about the children, not themselves.

Years later, I can still say that things are moving slowly in Haiti, as they do in many countries that have a poor infrastructure, an unstable government, and a population that suffers from broken spirits and bodies. I expect it will be many years before we see significant changes overall, but the children we care for are not victims of the stagnant recovery typical of the country as a whole. They are progressing at a fast rate, remaining healthy and growing. While a few were outside the normal parameters we like to see, we identified them and began efforts to begin moving them into the fold, and we quickly saw that the effort was paying off. We had achieved sustainability, which was leaving in place a process that offered the possibility of a long life, both physically and spiritually.

Jesus told the parable of the sower. The sower threw out seed, and some landed on the path, while other seed fell among thorns and rocky soil. Some seed, however, fell in fertile soil and yielded a rich crop. It was this last category that represented people who received the word of God and its many blessings and continued to grow without falling away. That is always our goal, and it's what we saw in Haiti: sustainability and growth that continues long after we have handed out medicine or counseled and prayed with our children and patients. We'd been to many countries, and the harvest was continuing to grow in rich soil that was sustaining our children.

We'll no doubt go back to Haiti many times in the future, but in 2011 we were bound for Ethiopia and Bangladesh. There was still so much to do in so many places.

Chapter Twenty-five
Our Daily Bread

We traveled to southern Bangladesh in October of 2011. It was going to be a challenging mission since many children in the impoverished country had never seen a doctor before, but getting there proved to be a task in itself. We left Phoenix for Chicago, picked up the rest of the team of twenty-one, left Chicago for Abu Dhabi, and drained the fuel tanks of the plane due to head winds. Next, we stopped in Kuwait to refuel, got to Abu Dhabi late, missed our connecting flight to Dhaka, and got a flight to Karachi, Pakistan, in order to catch a different flight to Dhaka. We could have stayed in Kuwait overnight, but that didn't sound very appetizing. We finally got to Karachi, but the connecting flight to Dhaka was delayed, necessitating a ten-hour wait in a Karachi transit area. It was tedious, to say the least. We finally arrived in Dhaka after leaving Phoenix forty-two hours earlier. To say we'd taken the scenic route would be an understatement. Strong headwinds across the northern hemisphere had slowed us done considerably, bucking us from left to right and up and down, eating up our fuel. We claimed all of our luggage, but fifteen boxes of meds and supplies (almost 800 pounds of needed stuff) didn't make it. The team spent the night in Dhaka, leaving early the next morning for a six-hour drive to the first clinic with whatever supplies they had in their personal bags, such as stethoscopes and blood pressure cuffs. They were going to run the first clinic as best they could, with no one knowing how it would go without a full complement of supplies.

Meanwhile, I stayed in Dhaka, waiting to see if the meds had made it in on the next flight. It was anxiety provoking, especially after such a long and bumpy journey. The medication finally arrived, and I made an eight-hour drive to the south of Bangladesh to catch up with the team late that night. God intervened when necessary and made it all work. He had our back despite one of the longest, most arduous trips we'd made to a region.

Jesus sent seventy-two disciples out to the villages he would visit, ordering them not to take a staff, sandals, or a traveler's sack. What they would need—including food and lodging—would be provided by the Holy Spirit. Our teams, of course, must take the necessary provisions to minister to the sick, but in a larger sense, we take only ourselves and a trust in Him each time we board a plane for a foreign land. We, too, must rely on the Holy Spirit to provide the strength, faith, and resolve that is needed for work in all of our clinics. At times, He even gives us supplies and helps us get past checkpoints and bureaucratic tangles, for we can never completely envision what need might pop up thousands of miles from home. He does not always give us what we ask for, but He never fails to give us what we need. Bangladesh posed a great many challenges before we could even get the operation off the ground, but we were not deterred, for we knew that God was orchestrating matters behind the scenes. Delays, missed flights, low fuel, headwinds—these were nothing for Him.

After the meds arrived, we all united in Khulna, ready to run the clinics and care for the children.

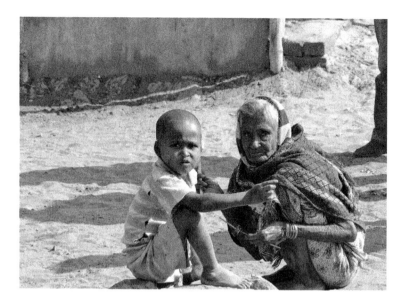

Chalna project was an isolated community that hadn't seen medical care in over fifteen years. Not surprisingly, the children were malnourished and sickly, but all laughed and smiled nevertheless. Prayer was the order of the day for the children—and us as well.

A Hindu woman came to Christ; others heard of the conversion and, in their curiosity, wondered if we really were who we said we were—His servants—for Bangladesh is primarily a Muslim country. We did our best to live up to the designation. We served 200 medical patients and nineteen dental patients with our usual emphasis on public health education, hygiene, water filtration systems, first aid training, and nutritional assessments. It was all done simultaneously, the team taking on all facets of health intervention and training—a ballet of sorts, with one continuous act and an encore. We had gone to a village and within six hours had left the inhabitants with a chance for a better life. Moving into a village with such a multi-faceted agenda is a bold, ambitious undertaking, but it worked because our teams are well trained and know how to choreograph the ballet perfectly. They were also led by the one who sent us there in the first place. It's good to know that He is always looking over our shoulders, whether on the best of days or the worst.

As mentioned, Bangladesh is a predominantly Muslim country, and we shared our message of God's love and good news but without force, coercion or stipulations. Some listened, some accepted, and some walked away. We encountered a woman with three husbands (one of whom beat her), a mother of a young girl with a heart defect, and the mother of a child with disabilities. If these cases sound daunting, they were, but it's what we expect when we travel down the back roads of the third world, especially where the population hasn't seen a physician in years. There are days when we find everyone generally happy and in decent condition except for malnutrition and routine illnesses that one might encounter anywhere—days when everything hums along smoothly, as when we breezed through clinics in Haiti and found little cholera—and days that test our limits and our patience. We mount our missions because we know people are hurting. There are complicated and dysfunctional family situations, including domestic abuse. And there are cases that reduce us to tears, such as those of Samnang or Pastor, but we have both weapons and shields to carry us through, for where two or more are gathered in His name, He is there in our midst. This is something that I've mentioned before, but it can't be emphasized enough. We are always in complete agreement that God Himself is present in the camps and in the hearts of the patients we see. He is always standing next to the exam tables, the dentist chairs, the pharmacy, and the counselors. Some might say that we are foolish for believing so and that our technical skills are the reason for our success. So be it. If we are fools, then we are fools for Christ.

The next clinic was the smoothest we'd ever experienced. We drove a short hour to Jogipol, where the pastor had the clinic set up and ready to go. Individual exam cubbies were waiting for doctors, nurses, healthcare workers, and patients. The children came, and we examined, treated, and cared for them. The most exceptional part of the visit was that two weeks prior to our arrival, the leadership of the project and church had met and prayed for a water filtration system. They didn't know we were bringing anything that remotely resembled what they were asking for since they had no idea of the full range of the supplies we bring to a given area. We pulled out the filtration system, attached it to a huge drum, and filtered water that was pure as any in the United States. Are prayers answered? You decide. I already know the answer.

It was a good day, and we next drove two hours to a remote village where we spent the day seeing 200 children and a fair number of adults. Medical, dental, water filtration, public health education, and first aid training were all performed under the sun. The heat was unbearable, with no wind and only marginal relief provided by some shade. A large Muslim population led by an imam was wary of us at first, but opened up to exams as the day grew on. Ironically, they grew increasingly anxious as the time approached for us to leave, knowing that many who had been waiting would not be seen. It's difficult to say "No more patients" today since the children were malnourished, sickly, tired, and lacked any semblance of even a single happy emotion. I looked at their faces and realized how little they had to be joyous about. We think we have it bad sometimes, but I wonder how much the average westerner could take if he or she had to live as these people did. Probably not much.

So the question I posed was this: just how bad did it have to get before people threw in the towel and said, "I give up"? From what I saw today, there were an awful lot of people who had thrown in the towel a long time ago, accepted the hand that had been dealt them, and learned to live with what they had, which was virtually nothing. Did we make a difference at the end of this particular day? I think we did, but not so much by giving them medication, pulling teeth, bringing in water filtration, or by teaching them first aid. What we did was validate them as worthy of being recognized as human beings— worthy of being loved, cared for, and given a sense of dignity. One person even said as much—the mother of a disabled child knew that we couldn't do much for him. He had a small head, injured brain, and was unable to walk or sit. But the smile he gave us when we reached out to him and held him without shying away from his inadequacies gave his mother validation as to how well she was caring for him and how much he meant to her.

It also showed how much the people of Bangladesh meant to *us*, for they reminded us that we don't really have it that bad, even on our worst days. When the people of Israel wandered in the desert on their way to the Promised Land, they complained about their lack of food. God sent them manna to collect in the morning, but the Israelites persisted in their complaints, demanding meat. God caused a wind to blow quail into the camps, and the people still grumbled. Generations later, Jesus suggested that people take a different approach to their needs by making a much simpler prayer: Give us our daily bread.

That's really all the people in the third world are asking for:

daily bread. Regardless of their environment—inner city, slum, or bush—they live in a desert in which they must scrape out a living or sometimes just subsist while waiting for help. For them, daily bread is a feast, a gift from God that gives them joy and optimism. That's why there are so many smiles surrounding the Medical Mercy teams at each and every clinic. We are their manna; we are their quails. We are the daily bread that God, in His goodness, has brought as if from nowhere.

Sadly, this mindset of thanksgiving in countries such as Haiti or Bangladesh isn't present in developed countries, where daily needs are taken for granted. But then tragedy strikes, such as a hurricane, tornado, mudslide, or wildfire, and everything is gone. Suddenly, the third world is right where a living room used to be. So here's the trick: live with a spirit of gratitude every day of the year, thankful for whatever you have, be it a little or a lot. It's the way most of the world's population lives twenty-four seven.

Nine thousand miles and a left turn east from Phoenix is where we were for a week—Bangladesh, a Muslim country, one of the poorest in the world. Almost twenty-five percent of the children were under five years of age, never making it to their sixth birthday. The average daily income for the working poor was two dollars a day. And the trip was harder than most. While getting to Dhaka on the last day of clinics, four of the six vans we had broke down during the ten-hour road trip from Khulna. We don't glide down three lane interstates; rather, we usually slog along ruts cutting through mud and dust and poor infrastructures.

Cultural differences, however, pose even greater challenges. When we're in a country with values different from ours, we begin to understand our purpose: to serve, to be humble, and to be compassionate. We were in a village where the imam came and chose to sit with his entourage to observe the activities of our medical team. He had the power to make trouble for us—or not. I introduced myself, spoke with him, and we exchanged blessings. His blessing to me was Mohammed-based, and mine to him was Christ-based. We smiled at each other as we clasped hands and then touched our hands to our hearts. There was mutual respect, understanding, and acceptance for who we were in God's eyes. He saw the children praying and how we cared for them. Later, he came to me and offered a heartfelt "Thank you." I couldn't have asked for anything more. Perhaps he saw what we did as a reflection of who we are and saw our purpose, which was to serve. Perhaps he even saw the will of God at work, the God who sends us around the world on His behalf. If that's what the imam saw, perhaps it was because we, too, saw what we were supposed to see: children who were vulnerable, hungry, poor, and at times forgotten, looking for a place in the world to experience life.

We gave the children their daily bread. Hopefully we gave the imam spiritual food as well. We certainly tried, but with a spirit of humility lest pride try to whisper to our minds that we have all the answers. We are painfully aware that we don't, but the best ambassador of the Gospel is action, letting good works speak for themselves, and the imam seemed receptive to our service to his people.

The team received its daily bread as well. When we give, it always comes back, and though some border crossings are more difficult than others, and though some clinics and patients leave us drained, we reap what we sow. On the long trip back to Phoenix, I knew we had given love, which is its own reward. It's daily bread.

Chapter Twenty-six
What Is Left Behind

It was January of 2012, and with God's grace it would be another year in which Medical Mercy would mount trips to take care of God's little ones, to reach out to those who have no names in the eyes of the world. It would be another year of performing our special brand of magic, which is making the invisible appear in their villages to become citizens of a world that cared they existed.

Next stop? India. We were headed to the southern part of coastal India off the Bay of Bengal. We would be based in the small town of Puri. With a population of 150,000, Puri is well known as a pilgrimage site for Hindus, who have a pantheon of thousands of gods and goddesses. One might think that it is pure folly to engage in counseling and pastoral care in countries that are not Christian in identity, but the mission Christ issued was to preach the Gospel to the whole world, not just the suburbs of an affluent country. We therefore take our medicine and our message to the far corners of the globe, proclaiming it and then stepping back spiritually to let the Holy Spirit do its work. We know details such as blood pressure, lab results, heart rate, and a multitude of symptoms, but God knows the hearts of those we encounter. That is what keeps us humble.

       ⁓⁓⁓

We've all heard the saying "What are we bringing to the table?" when we talk about negotiations and relationships. In other words, what is it that we bring that will be valuable to another person? In the case of Medical Mercy, it's obvious. We bring medical care, prayer, and all of the other services I've described thus far. But here's where I like to go a little off-script in what I have alluded to above, namely the command that has been given to us to take the Gospel message to the world. I am always aware of what we bring, but I am more acutely aware of that which we leave behind, such as memories, interactions, changed lives, and the improvement of what is often the drab, hopeless existence of those we meet. It is always my hope that we leave behind the power of prayer, the introduction to a God who is singular in His reign, and at times new believers, individuals who have come to Christ and seen a different spiritual dimension open up before their eyes. What we leave behind is an important consideration since the day always comes for us step aboard a plane and leave those we love thousands of miles in our wake.

     I am often reminded of Jesus' parable of the talents, which was a denomination of currency in Judea two thousand years ago. A master embarked upon a trip, giving five talents to a servant to manage affairs in his absence. To another servant he gave two talents, and yet another received one talent. Upon his return, the master asked for an accounting from his servants. The first servant had doubled the talents, yielding ten. The second had also doubled what had been entrusted to him, yielding four. The third, however, had buried the talent to ensure that he wouldn't lose it, afraid of his master's reputation as a hard businessman.

In my own life, I see two applications for the parable. I am expected to multiply the gifts I am given and make a greater return to God, for scripture also says that from the person who has been given much, much will be expected. By the same token, I continually hope and pray that what we leave behind—what we entrust to those we have treated and prayed with—will likewise be increased in our absence. A great example is how Pastor Daniel took the Heimlich Maneuver and passed it on to others, who actually used it to save lives. And then there were the people in Haiti who had practiced all of the preventative measures to stop further cases of cholera. We are entrusted with talents—pun intended—that we, in turn, entrust to others. It's the way the kingdom of God spreads.

Sometimes we're focused on the big picture and lose sight of the details. Day one of our clinic at the village of Orissa represented the big picture. We set in motion a medical clinic, with both old and new team members getting into the swing of things very quickly due to the incredible pre-planning of the Indian support staff. A total of fifty people kept our three-track system running smoothly. That was the big picture.

Stunting—when a child's height does not match his or her age on the growth chart—affects over millions of children in India. An Indian boy thirteen, is one of the millions whose growth is severely stunted. Could we help him? Not in the sense of getting him to grow anymore, but what we did was to assure him that, despite his size, he was as valuable a member of the community as anybody else. He smiled and became animated because he realized that he could be part of "the big picture." It is said the least on earth shall be the greatest in the Kingdom of God, but our mission is to affirm the dignity of children such as this stunted Indian boy so that he realizes that, right here and right now, he does not have to be ashamed of who he is.

Sadly, there are many other serious health concerns besides stunting. Polio, for example, is still prevalent in India despite the availability of vaccines. Poor compliance with vaccination protocols and a lack of awareness and education about the disease yielded what we saw, which was children wearing old-style, bulky braces, heavy and uncomfortable, worn for life. Also, there was no physical therapy available for people with the disease. A girl with polio asked if there was a way to make her leg stronger, but the hard answer was no. What we did instead was to make her life more comfortable by getting her a new brace, one that was lightweight, comfortable, and less obtrusive. It was yet another instance where all we could do was lessen the existing damage since preventive measures available in most of the world weren't on the radar of the population we were dealing with. Lessening pain, however, is better than ignoring it altogether, and therein lies our mantra for so many: we do what we can. More importantly, though, we noticed the detail hidden in the bigger picture: the girl's braces were cumbersome and painful. She needed relief. The stunted boy and the girl with polio were real people camouflaged by tens of millions of other people suffering and in need. If we were going to be good stewards, something had to be left behind for them as well.

The big picture was clear for Bangladesh. There were many children who needed care. It was the details of the picture, the areas that were difficult to see unless one focused a little sharper, that Medical Mercy was looking for. Individuals rather than population numbers and statistics. We remain focused for the rest of the week, looking closely at those who came to the clinics. Our eyes were strained, but our hearts were filled.

∽ゐⓒ∾

Rule of thumb for Medical Mercy: expect the unexpected. Plan for the worst and hope for the best. Most days throw us the proverbial curve ball, and that's what the next day at Orissa was like. The flow of the clinic was the same, but the patients were smaller in stature than the day before, a little sicker, and their stories were far from the norm even by Medical Mercy's standards. While many children were hugged, sung to, and prayed with, it was the unexpected encounter—the worst case scenario—that put the day into perspective. Three children stood out. One child had a single but serious complaint, which was that he was depressed. He lived in a boarding house for children who were single or double orphans, meaning that one or both parents had died. One day he had received a letter addressed to him saying that his father had died recently. It came out of the blue, leaving him devastated.

Another child carried with him a picture of his parents that had been taken a while back. He was ten years old. He showed me the picture and asked if I had seen them or knew anything about them since he hadn't seen them in five years. How sad that a child was still searching, hoping against hope, for his missing parents after so long a period of time. He woke up one day and they were both gone. He'd lived in the street until he found a home in the village, having been taken in by a kind family. I looked at the picture and couldn't find any words to say. I simply shook my head no. He responded by shaking his head as well and then silently cried. I hugged him and prayed with him—it was all I could do. He left the clinic, the picture still clutched in his hand.

The third child was six years old. I asked her if I could take her picture and show it to others so I could witness that she was as much a child to be valued and recognized as any other. She was hesitant at first, but then said yes. Burned by falling into a pot of boiling water at the age of three, her skin was mottled, a combination of black and brown pigment, and her pink lower lip drooped. She told me that she wouldn't look in the mirror because of the accident that left her scarred. She was the daughter of a fisherman and his wife, the lowest class of the caste system in the region—poorer than poor. She was not a sponsored child, just one of the children in the village who came to us for medical care. I knew that if she wasn't embraced and surrounded by a loving community, she would be lost to the world, never marrying and always the subject of ridicule. She would likely be taken advantage of and perhaps even take her life at some point in the future. We had a vision to care for such children, and she became one of them. I was humbled to become part of her life from then on.

We had been holding clinics in a fishing village in the town of Puri, from which many of the children came. The village had a population of 25,000 and was considered the poorest of the environs of Puri. What spoke to me the next day was a story told by Pastor David. Thirty-nine years earlier he was an alcoholic, a hit man for a mobster organization, and a worshipper of an Indian monkey god, the image of which was tattooed on his arm. He fell off his bike one day after drinking too much and woke up to find a piece of paper next to him with a scripture verse on it that said, "Jesus is God." He wondered who this man could be who claimed to be god when so many other gods were worshipped in India, such as the monkey god. Pastor David went to a church the next morning and the day after that. In fact, he went to church for the next 365 days, studying the bible until he found the way. He began pastoring in the fishing village, and by the time we arrived he had a congregation of over 900 people. He tended to the One Child Matters children and served with us while we were there. What was it that made him change? He himself couldn't really put his finger on it, but he did say one thing that touched me: "A monkey god is simply that—a monkey god. But Jesus is a god who became man, someone who came to earth to carry our sins. How could I not believe in that?" He spoke these words in broken English as the children ran and played around us. He looked at them and quietly said, "They, too, will one day hopefully see that the monkey is just a monkey." I took his hand, and we prayed together as the children continued to play. He was determined to leave something of himself behind in the years ahead. He wanted to multiply the faith that had been given to him by a master who expects a return on His investment.

Something seemed to be out of sorts. We finished up the last two days of clinics, but we were feeling lost, not because of what we weren't able to accomplish, but because we couldn't do more. The last day of clinic was probably the main reason for this odd feeling that things remained incomplete. On Thursday we had seen patients as we always do, none with unusual complaints, and then Friday came. About an hour's drive from Puri was a small parcel of land where 900 children were malnourished, sickly, and isolated—every last one of them. There was room for 370 children in the area's school, but the rest of them had nowhere to go. The village was one of displaced people of the lower caste, unwanted by the general population. They wanted for much but were given nothing. We came upon this place due to a change in plans—divine intervention perhaps—but it was good that we had. We all felt that we had to make the fishing village a priority, for there were further details hidden in the big picture, and we were compelled to leave something behind, something that might make a difference.

That, I suppose, was the deeper story of my trip to India. It is a large country with a burgeoning population in which people—mostly the children—become numbers instead of individuals who are loved and cared for. To help them, one has to focus one's inner sight differently. We've all seen pictures such as "Where's Waldo," in which a player has to find a familiar face hidden among dozens of others crowded together. We always endeavor not to gloss over anyone, for each individual has a special worth.

Jesus noticed details all the time. Once, he was walking through a small village called Nain. He saw a funeral procession in which a widow was walking beside her son's bier as the townspeople took him to be buried. Such a sight was common since infant mortality—and mortality in general—was very high. Women had several children since thirty to fifty percent never made it out of their teens, but the widow of Nain had no others. Jesus stopped the funeral procession and approached the bier because he felt sorry for the widow, who had no one to help her or care for her. He brought the young man back to life and gave him to his mother. The procession was a common sight in Palestine, but it didn't go unnoticed by Jesus, who was concerned with everyone's intrinsic worth. When he moved on, he left behind life where there had been death, hope where there had been mourning.

That is what Medical Mercy always tries to do: remember that what's left behind is as important as what we bring.

Chapter Twenty-seven
The Fruits of Our Labor

In late February and early March of 2012 I traveled to three countries in five days: Honduras, Haiti, and the Dominican Republic. It was important to do follow-up care to ascertain just how well our sustainability was holding up. I expected that I would find a few hiccups here and there—things that would need some tweaking—since not everything in the United States healthcare system works perfectly either. If people fell through the cracks in America, it was safe to assume that there would be issues to address in these countries. St. Paul traveled to many cities in the ancient world—Colossus, Phillipi, Rome, Corinth, Thessolonika, Ephesus, and others—and his epistles to the Christian communities in these cities were written to take their spiritual pulse, to see if they were continuing to live a new life in Christ. St. Paul was a contemporary of Jesus, and the message he preached was quite new in the region and had to be safeguarded since false doctrine occasionally tried to creep in. He also received reports from various disciples who reported to him during his years of imprisonment. That's essentially what I was going to do: take the medical and spiritual temperature of these countries and see what was holding and what might need shoring up.

My impressions of what we'd accomplished on our missions

were very positive. Honduras had 3,000 One Child Matters children in over twenty projects, many of them in Tegucigalpa, some in the north and some in the south. But how do you ensure that all 3,000 children get consistent healthcare all of the time? The answer is that you have doctors like Victoria and Francisco, who were taking care of the One Child Matters children twenty-four hours a day. Victoria and Francisco were recent graduates from medical school in Honduras and had a calling in their hearts to minister to the underserved, to give everything and expect nothing and to be there for all who came to them. Through a series of events—and some divine intervention—One Child Matters came upon these two noble physicians, and our relationship with them was born. Victoria and Francisco visited all of the children multiple times a year and established a nutritional supplementation program, a twenty-four hour call center, an ambulance, a central clinic base, a mobile clinic program, and twice yearly physical exams for all the children. It was amazing! These two doctors had gone beyond what might be expected in many areas, and through their dedication, coupled with God's power, produced all of the extras cited above that went far beyond the presence of a single clinic.

St. Paul had many disciples to help him, such as Silas, Barnabas, and Timothy, among others, and here were modern-day disciples who were proving to be exemplary stewards. I was seeing the seeds we had planted now growing, their fruit going beyond our original efforts and expectations. It was God's doing, of course, but I was beginning to realize that miracles were happening. I knew in a direct way that God could indeed do more than what we ask for. In John 14:12, Jesus says, "I tell you the truth, anyone who believes in me will do the same works I have done, and even greater works, because I am going to be with the Father" (NLT). I was witnessing the greatness of God and the fruits of our labor—and His Spirit—right before my eyes.

In Haiti, I revisited Dubuisson and saw that it had grown and that the community had settled into a place ripe for expansion. While some of the children were malnourished, anemic, and had pneumonia, I came across one area that One Child Matters and a partner U.S. church were looking to embrace. The church had no roof on it, but it was to become the center of a One Child Matters Child Development Center for one hundred children. Haiti had been hit hard by the earthquake and the cholera outbreak, but even in such a devastated country seeds were sprouting through the ashes of disaster. How was such a thing possible without the hand of God directing events?

At the end of my stay in Haiti, I'd wanted to hear that all was well and that all the children were healthy, growing, strong, and without illness. We weren't there yet, but we were moving in the right direction. The children were well-cared for physically, spiritually and emotionally. They were holding their own, getting vitamins and meals, and when they got sick, they were taken to a local clinic. There were bumps in the road, but nothing we couldn't smooth out.

In communities in the Dominican Republic, children found themselves at small grocery stores, seeking a candy bar or a soft drink. The question was how they could do this without any money. The answer was that they begged, and I saw two boys doing just that. Even from far away, I could sense that the shopkeeper, barely keeping his little store open with a few patrons, was giving in to them. They both left with a small piece of candy, a gift from one who had little to give. This kind of scene set the tone for all that I saw in the Dominican Republic as I moved from one project to another. The staff was gifting from their hearts, using personal funds and resources to help children in addition to those from One Child Matters.

This was the case with a twelve-year-old girl. A few months earlier she was taken ill with an unknown infection, became combative, and lost consciousness. The project leader took her to the hospital and, before even asking One Child Matters for help, put down a sizable amount of money from her own pocket and that of the other project staff to get the care the girl needed immediately. The girl spent two weeks in the hospital, slowly recovering. I saw her CT scan and her EEG, and an area of infection was clearly noticeable in her brain. The project director and her staff prayed for her continually and also made sure that funds were available for the care the girl needed on a daily basis. Little was done in government hospitals in the Dominican Republic unless one paid up front for medications, and I saw the bill for diapers, IV solutions, medications, and more. All of these expenses were paid for by the project staff. The little girl left the hospital with some mild residual neurological changes, but she was recovering more and more of her function on a daily basis. I examined her, and she was bright, happy, and thankful for her life. She gave me permission to share her story in order to say "Thank you" to all who had cared for her.

I'd come to assess the healthcare programs we'd put in place in the Dominican Republic, Honduras, and Haiti. I was struck with the fact that the programs were not only working well, but that they were also being expanded by the projects themselves thanks to a high degree of self-direction and a lot of effort. Most of all, I was struck with the kindness of the One Child Matters staff. To save a child's life is a heart-driven act that no formal program can ever match. And isn't that what we're all about? To ensure that all children have an opportunity to experience his or her God-given potential?

We had apparently done far more than I realized, or should I say that God had exceeded our expectations? The fruits of our labor were in plain evidence. We had planted seed and taught people to fish for themselves so that they could become self-sufficient. The healthcare worker program I'd developed seven years earlier was ensuring that healthcare would be ongoing in Haiti, Ethiopia, Cambodia and Swaziland, but what about Kenya?

There was no need to worry. The healthcare workers there were sharp, inquisitive, and motivated when I checked in. With eleven projects in the country and nine well-trained healthcare workers, referrals were down by fifty-five percent. Additionally, healthcare costs for the projects were down fifty percent, and each healthcare worker was seeing ten children a month. Finally, thirty-two children with life-threatening illnesses had been treated but not hospitalized, signaling the competency and professionalism of each worker.

Joyce was a perfect example of a dedicated Medical Mercy healthcare worker. Working near Malindi, she had set up her clinic with medications and a little table. Her fanny pack was her doctor's bag, with a stethoscope, blood pressure cuff, and all the tools she needed to do a comprehensive physical examination. She was saving lives with just the basics, but with love as her main medicine, she was working wonders.

God was working miracles. It was another case of the mustard seed—the smallest of all seeds, as Jesus said—growing while we weren't looking. But this realization almost begs the question of "How was it happening?"

While I don't have any definitive answer, I do think the most obvious conclusion is rooted in love. It says in 1 Corinthians 13 that "Love is patient, love is kind. It does not envy, it does not boast, it is not proud. It does not dishonor others, it is not self-seeking, it is not easily angered, it keeps no record of wrongs. Love does not delight in evil but rejoices with the truth. It always protects, always trusts, always hopes, always perseveres" (NIV). It would be easy to judge people we see of another faith, but we accept them for who they are. If someone has faltered badly in his her personal life, we don't judge, blame, or dishonor. We listen, pray, and do what we can to help the person, for as St. Paul says in the above quote, this attitude is the very heart of love. When we approach a project of hurting people with agape love, the rest takes care of itself in ways that can't always be explained.

But even this represents only a partial explanation. The love experienced by the people we encounter ultimately comes from God, for all of scripture tells us that His very essence is love. It is his will to draw all men and women to Himself and to bind the wounds of those who have been hurt and scarred, whether physically, emotionally, or spiritually. The Book of Revelation says that at the end of time Christ will be joined to His church—His body of believers—in what scripture calls "the wedding feast of the lamb."

In the Gospel of Luke, Jesus told the parable of a feast. A man gave a great banquet, but the invited guests made excuses and didn't go. The man told his servants to invite the poor, the lame, the crippled, and the blind. They did and reported that there was still room in the banquet hall. The man then instructed his servants to go to the open roads and hedgerows and collect anyone they could find so that his hall would be filled.

I took a step back from my travels, assessments, and follow-ups, in awe of what I was seeing. Before my eyes, in slums and villages far from what most people call civilization, there were God's little ones—the poor, lame, crippled, abused, wounded, and broken. He was inviting the homeless, the rag pickers, the maimed, the depressed, the orphans, and all those whose stories had moved me to tears, people who had no hope or means of getting well. And, of course, the children, who were so close to the heart of Jesus. God was calling everyone to participate in His life and, one day, the wedding feast of the lamb. For me, it was a moment of profound humility, almost like missing the forest for the trees, as I realized that I was witnessing the gathering of God's people through an outpouring of love—His and ours. It's not something I could see when standing in the heat or rain or mud while conducting exams, but this gathering was also a big picture made up of many details. The power of God's love was in the process of creating His kingdom, and His miracles were real and they were happening in the twenty-first century.

I think that these follow-up trips were another tap on the shoulder from Him, much like the ones I received as a youth. He was telling me that my teams and I were moving in the right direction. All I could say was, "Thank you."

Chapter Twenty-Eight
Feeding His Sheep

It was May of 2012, the rainy season in Kenya, when rivers flood and washes overflow. Our team was there, and we walked across a wash but had to take all our meds over in a small truck. With no four-wheel drive, the vehicle required a lot of pulling and pushing, but it made it across okay. We were headed to a small village called Kiburro, and it took us two hours to go the thirty miles, which was an indication of how deep in the bush we were. This was Masai territory, traditional in dress and culture. Women wore beaded jewelry, men leapt about with long sticks and machetes, and there was much rhythmic dancing. We were greeted with such displays and blessed with them when we left.

I paused to look about from where we were holding clinic and could see the valleys of the Masai territory in every direction. Umbrella trees gave shade to acres of bush and then open plains. We saw gazelle roaming freely and small herds of goats herded under the watchful eyes of young Masai boys. Having grown up in Somalia, Kenya brought back many memories. I felt at home. I was fulfilling a dream of being a doctor and practicing in east Africa, where the impulse had first originated. I was six years old when I made that my goal, and there I was, still observing just as Mahmoud had taught me to do, searching for the details in the bigger picture. Perhaps that's why I saw not just a drought, but thirst in the mouths of small children. I didn't just see the colorful dress and beads of the Masai, but people who had souls that God cherished and longed to embrace in a deeper way. I didn't see a remote population likely to show up on a National Geographic special, but rather a group of people with specific needs. The details inside the big picture—their names and faces and struggles—were there.

We saw all of the One Child Matters children—and then some. The healthcare workers shone brightly as they examined the children, their skills fine-tuned under the guidance of the U.S. team. As usual, the One Child Matters children were much healthier than the non-sponsored children in the village, a continued testimony to the healthcare worker program. Perhaps one day we would have all of the children of Kiburro under our wing.

It was another day in the bush at a small Masai community called Olootepes, a population unknown to most due to the nomadic nature of the Masai. I learned that the drought season there was dismal. Children got one cup of water a day, if that. The river beds were dry, and I was told that when it finally rained, the river water was dirty and undrinkable. We were so far into the bush that trucking water in from the nearest town would cost $250, not including the cost for the 500 gallons of water. I wondered how the people survived. One Child Matters fed the children there, and they drank from the sources put in place. It helped somewhat, but more needed to be done. Water filtration systems only work when there's a source of water to begin with.

Atop a mesa, surrounded by the plains of the Rift Valley, we worked side by side with the healthcare workers examining the children and some of the adults. It was all worth it. Far away from what we knew as home, it still felt right. What we needed, however, was to have the water flow so that the children could drink. We had only one method only at our disposal: prayer.

Many people ask if Medical Mercy is simply a Band-Aid, a feel good medical team going in and doing a song and dance routine before leaving for our comfortable surroundings back home. These are hard words, but they're asked all the same. As I already indicated, nothing could be further from the truth since Medical Mercy aims for sustainability in every region in which we operate. But when we were in the very remote bush in Kenya, perhaps it was a legitimate question if someone wasn't familiar with our work. Not surprisingly, my answer to critics is faith-based and appeals to the *permanent* presence of God in all situations, which I believe is analogous to the continued presence of One Child Matters in our projects. I recalled Psalm 139, which seemed appropriate for the region, as well as many others we visit that are isolated and off the grid—but not God's.

> Where could I go from your Spirit?
> Where could I flee from your presence?
> If I go to the heavens you are there;
> If I make my bed in the depths you are there.
> If I say, "Surely the darkness will hide me
> And the light become night around me,"
> Even the darkness would not be dark to you;
> The night would shine like the day,
> For darkness is as light to you.
> (Psalm 139: 7-8; 11-12/JB)

If we were just applying Band-Aids, we wouldn't bother to travel to such remote regions, many off the beaten path. We do so, however, because we know that His people are there. Perhaps they are out of sight and out of mind for most, but not for us and not for God. As the above psalm implies, God is everywhere, and no one is beyond His sight. Other verses of the psalm say the following.

> If I rise on the wings of the dawn,
> if I settle on the far side of the sea,
> even there your hand will guide me,
> your right hand will hold me fast.
> (Psalm 139: 9-10/JB)

That's the key. God's hand guides our missions, and through our efforts, He never abandons those He cares for, those He signals out for treatment by Medical Mercy, and no one is beyond His reach. He is a constant God, and since we act in His name, we make sure that we keep in touch with the clinics and centers we establish, which is why I check back with our projects on a regular basis. God is present everywhere and to everyone, and the notion of a band-aid approach to health-care is alien to covenant relationships. Our intention, there-fore, is to be ever-present to those we serve as God Himself is ever-present to His people.

And that was our approach in Kenya. We left behind an infrastructure in healthcare. We'd identified the moderately or severely malnourished, conducted our usual nutritional assess-ments, and put in place a concrete follow-up program, includ-ing referrals for children who needed additional care.

Isn't this what Jesus did before ascending to heaven? He'd accomplished his primary mission. He'd taught, forgiven sins, and healed thousands. After his resurrection, however, he gave explicit instructions to his disciples to carry on His ministry. They were to continue to remember Him around a communal meal. They were to pray always, forgive sins in His name, and minister to the poor and sick. In fact, three times He told Peter, who was designated as the leader of the twelve, to "Feed my sheep" (John 21:17/JB). In short, they were to maintain a continued presence of gospel values. But Jesus knew that they couldn't do this alone. He left a permanent presence with His followers by sending them the Holy Spirit, the Advocate. That's what I call the ultimate follow-up care.

I firmly believe that the same Holy Spirit is alive today, still moving, healing, and bringing the Father's love to all who would receive it. This was my epiphany when I saw how things were running smoothly in the countries we served. Miracles were happening and God's kingdom was growing. As I left Kenya, I felt certain that we had not only accomplished our goals, but that His presence and power remained behind.

We'd gone deep into the bush. To paraphrase the psalm, He was there, too.

Chapter Twenty-nine

The Right Place
at the Right Time

Just when we think that everything is in place, the ground shakes and it all tumbles over. Such was the case with our well-intentioned plans to go to Zimbabwe. It was October of 2012, and after planning for a year, accumulating stacks of credentials from the medical folk who were going, writing over 200 emails (yes, I counted them), and a lot of behind the scenes work from a group of dedicated, tireless, and uncomplaining partners on the ground in Zimbabwe, it all went for naught in a matter of days. Approval from those who would credential us to practice medicine in Zimbabwe was not to be. The new plan? Swaziland. It took just three days to pull it all together, with our partners in Swaziland agreeing to welcome us and make flight changes and arrange hotel accommodations. Everything was in place—same goals, different venue—but I notified the team so that they could decide if the change in our destination would alter their heart for going. Nope, it didn't, so off we went to Swaziland to visit five projects in one week. I planned to travel to Zimbabwe and Mozambique after Swaziland to see if there had been a change in heart so that we'd have an opportunity to help the children there. For the time being, however, we were ready to gear up and plant more seed.

There was no internet service, so all of my communications once we arrived occurred thanks to my Blackberry, but there was a great deal to share since we went to work right out the gate. We went to the very first project ever opened, a medical clinic established five years earlier. We saw sick children, one who was sent to a hospital. Another child had suffered from severe neurological devastation from birth, and yet a third needed her foot amputated due to progressive gangrene. All of this happened in addition to five hours of lectures to health-care workers and our customary nutritional assessments, dental exams, spiritual counseling, and dispensing of medication. All patients were entered into our database using bar codes, and reading glasses were made available for the elderly and others in need. This was medicine and covenant care at warp speed, but the team didn't blink an eye. For Medical Mercy professionals who "know the flow," many patients can be seen in a short time without compromising accuracy, professionalism, or pastoral care. Love is the best kind of spiritual adrenaline there is.

Day two found us at a place far from the main city, a small project with 150 children. It was a somewhat slow day, allowing us to move through the patient load easily and with little stress. The children were anxious for attention, going from one of us to another, looking for and receiving hugs. We looked at their faces as they sang and expressed happiness despite the lack of comforts as we knew them, and I wondered if we should look at ourselves once in a while to see if we truly need all that we have. There was a hunger in these children that went beyond the desire for more food. It was a spiritual hunger, a desire for someone to look at them and say, "Yes! I see and love you! I know you're there!" That's all any of us really needs at the level of spirit.

But every day is different. Day three gave us rain, and a lot of it. We were in a remote area, working under a big tent, when the heavens opened and thunder boomed. There was also lightening, and metal poles were no longer our friends. We collapsed the tent, ran for shelter, and kept seeing patients using flashlights in a crowded room. It was a classic case of making lemons out of lemonade. It was especially cramped, with a hundred people crowding in for care. Somehow we did it.

Day four saw us return to Mbabane, the small project isolated on the border of Swaziland and Mozambique. Rain continued to disrupt the orderly flow of children in the clinic, but we managed. The children were well cared for, but there was a need for a lot more. Barefoot, cold, and in tattered clothes, they came for the meal that sustained them for another day, plus a night of sleep. It occurred to me that a billion dollars is spent on a presidential campaign, most of which is donated money, but what an enormous difference that billion dollars could make in the lives of the children we see, or even in the lives of the many children who are homeless in the United States. Even a fraction of that amount could make a huge difference and provide meals, vaccinations, vitamins, and medical exams. These things are routinely available for most, but not all, in the United States, but in the third world, they can make the difference between life and death. So I come back to the same question: how much of what we have do we really need? A billion dollars is a lot of money. No one should be frowned upon for being successful or wealthy, but at a higher level, it's all about stewardship and what we do with what we've been given.

I saw the faces of children as they looked at me, and I wondered what they were thinking. The children didn't know anything about political campaigns or, for that matter, the affluent lifestyles of western civilization. Maybe that was a good thing since, as I already mentioned, people are rooted in their own time and culture. When we export our own technology and culture—they seem to go hand in hand these days—to the third world, are we not also exporting the potential for greed that accompanies these things. Just as a computer virus hides on hard drives, is there a spiritual virus hiding in our exports? I'm not sure. These are difficult questions, but I suppose the answer lies not in *what* we have but in how we use it. On this particular day, the children had what they needed the most, and I was satisfied that they seemed to know that we were there for them. That's the biggest export—the biggest contribution—anyone can make: being there for someone else. Being present when present. It's a pity that we can't make *that* a billion dollar campaign.

We did a final day in the rain, wind, and cold. The air buzzed with activity as we saw 150 patients in four hours. We'd seen 1,111 patients in five days, although many of the clinics started late or were cut short because of the weather. After all was said and done, however, we saw who we needed to see— and more. The team worked tirelessly, and we saw children with illnesses ranging from pneumonia to simple infections to complex illnesses. Some significant illnesses required referrals to advanced healthcare facilities.

There was one day when we came across children who had no shoes and no decent clothing. They shivered in the cold rain as team members took off their socks and gave them to the children, as well as shoes that had been brought by a team member. Even some of the clothing that we wore was given to children we thought should be better protected from the cold. The team members were servants beyond any title they might have had on the team. Our intended destination had been Zimbabwe, not Swaziland, but it turned out to be one of the most powerful missions we'd done in a long time. The children needed us, we needed them, and without the incredible help, guidance, and support from the Swaziland home team, we would not have been able to pull it off.

Doors open and doors close. It's not done by us but by God. For whatever reason, Swaziland was where we were supposed to be. This doesn't mean that Mozambique doesn't have a multitude of people who need our help, but we trust that the timing is what it is for a reason. Indeed, maybe that's the way it is for most things in life. Perhaps people, places, and things are put in our path for a reason. The next time you meet a stranger, find a book on a park bench, or learn that your flight has been delayed, consider that maybe it's for a reason. He knocks frequently, but we have to open the door.

Chapter Thirty

Reaching the Summit

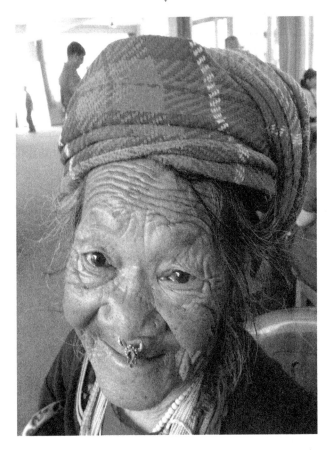

There are mountains and then there are mountains. We were in Nepal in April of 2013, and Mt. Everest loomed in the distance. It is a mountain that has claimed many lives but has given many more the satisfaction of beating it. A twenty-two-member U.S. team had been preparing for the climb, but Everest didn't beckon us to ascend, but rather to wonder in awe at its magnificence. It is truly one of the earth's majestic mountains and an example of the beauty of God's creation. It was the children who beckoned us, children cared for by loving teachers and pastors. We would hold five days of medical clinics in order to bring a sense of calm to the children and treat the illnesses they had. We made no pretense of being able to scale the mountain of sustainable healthcare and perfect nutritional growth just yet, but despite a few setbacks and roadblocks—even a slip or two down the side of our own mountain—we weren't worried. As the U.S. trekkers prepared to climb Everest, we would begin the climb of daily clinics, seeing as many children and adults as possible, going slowly, methodically, and carefully, taking each step with determination, comforted by the fact that we had the best guide we could have: God.

Sleep was elusive. I was in Kathmandu, my mind racing in the shadow of the mountain my team and I would be climbing. We arrived in Nepal after forty-eight hours of travel. We rested, got to know each other, and had fellowship and orientation, getting ready to start the climb. I asked the team to reflect on the question of why we conducted our missions. Many have asked me what Medical Mercy does and how we go about it, and those questions are easy enough to answer. But the question I am rarely asked was *why* we stage our clinics. Few really want to know. They are more interested in the what and the how, which are easier questions to get one's mind around. We treat disease, train healthcare workers, teach hygiene, counsel . . . and all the rest. I asked the team to reflect on the why so that they could be prepared to answer the question if ever asked. I had my own answer. It took a while to find, but it was there—solid, indisputable, non-negotiable, and personal. It was what gave me the strength to climb the mountain that week, a mountain of long days in clinics with sick children, at times frustrated because we couldn't climb higher. I decided to share my answer with the team at the end of the week and trusted that the team would share its own answers with me.

We were leaving in a few short hours for our "base camp." It was time to sleep, but before I closed my eyes, I spent a few minutes talking to someone who knew me and why I traveled with Medical Mercy. *He* was my answer.

When nothing happens out of the ordinary, it's easy to wonder if anything has gone wrong. And that's just what happened on our first day. It was probably the best day of clinics we'd ever had in all the trips we'd made. There was an easy setup and smooth flow through the clinic, with 200 patients seen with time to spare. There were a few glitches, such as no electricity, no generator, and therefore no power for the drills and power tools the dentists needed. They improvised all the same, and teeth got pulled, repaired, and cleaned, and all was good with the dental track. The children were relatively healthy, with a few falling outside the norm, but they were easily attended to and treated.

Several children caught our attention, however. A ten-year-old girl with a heart murmur was told she needed surgery at age two, but she hadn't received any follow-up on her condition. Now, eight years later, she asked if it was a good time to get the surgery done. The answer was no, it wouldn't happen—not today, not tomorrow, and not any time soon. Valve surgery requires an extensive workup as well as post-op care, and it wasn't something that could be handled on the fly. This is the tragedy when a potentially serious condition isn't addressed in a timely fashion. The girl's heart murmur was very fixable, but we couldn't do it in our clinic, and finding the time, place, and money in Nepal wasn't likely to happen.

A ten-year-old boy with a mechanical brace on his right leg showed up in a wheel chair. He'd been hit by a motorcycle a year earlier. Some type of surgery had been performed, and his leg had been put in a brace. Now, a year later, having not walked all this time, he asked us to fix it so that he could get out of his chair. The leg was misaligned—turned inward—and required a competent orthopedic surgeon to fix it. Out of the blue, an anesthesiologist who was the director of a nearby private hospital came for an unannounced visit and offered to have an orthopedic surgeon see the child at no cost. Miracles can happen in many ways, and I had no doubt that the appearance of the anesthesiologist was no accident.

We'd started the climb and were a few hundred feet up the mountain, where we stayed until the following day, when it would again be time to serve those who He sent to us.

The rising sun brought those who were going to the base camp on Mt. Everest to a gathering place where they awaited their ride. They would have to climb 17,500 feet, which they would do in four to six days depending on their strength and endurance. They would spend another ten days to two weeks at the base camp, getting acclimated to the altitude in preparation for the trek to the 29,300 feet summit. Their strategy was to wait for a window of opportunity—a break in the weather—since they had only two weeks to get up and back. I was in awe of their fortitude and determination.

At the same time, those of us who were going to a project to hold our medical clinic gathered in a place to await our ride as well. We had a thirty-minute ride to the project, a full day of clinic, saw children a little sicker than we saw yesterday, and I was in awe of our own team's fortitude and determination. The climbers and the Medical Mercy team had two very different destinations and goals. My team acclimated not to altitude, but to the poverty that we witnessed, the malnourished children, and the sense of hopelessness that covered the faces of mothers who couldn't care for their children. We approached our base camp no differently than the trekkers. Our steps were deliberate as we made sure every action counted in order to reach our goal. That was *our* trek.

We walked half a mile into the project, carrying all of our supplies without benefit of sherpas. We treated children with asthma, pneumonias, and ear infections. We saw children who were stunted and short for their age as a result of being malnourished. Those children would be vulnerable to chronic illnesses and a short life span. Our sponsored children were given a chance to reach the summit, a summit symbolized by making a life out of nothing and being able to breathe without coughing and wheezing.

Nepal is a beautiful country. The children were uniquely beautiful, with facial features and smiles that radiated love. I slept a few hours and waited for the rising sun. In the morning, we gathered to trek to the next project—a few thousand feet higher and closer to the top, which was healthcare for those who needed it the most.

There are times when life brings us joyous moments despite the hardships we face. I saw a letter written by a young man who had been sponsored for the previous thirteen years.

Dear Sponsor,

I am eighteen years old and live in Nepal. You have sponsored me since I was five years old. Many things have happened in my life since you chose to help support me.

I now know Jesus, I am about to graduate and go on to college in computer science, and I now volunteer [and] teach computers at my school. None of this would have happened were it not for God using you to help in my life.

I want you to know that I have kept every letter and card you have ever sent me. What you have sent, I will treasure for a lifetime. The best was that you gave so that I could be a man. You have prayed for me and even sent clothes for my mother. I keep your photos and pray for you.

You see, my mom is my only parent. We are very poor, and she works in a hotel making just enough to pay our rent and food. What you have done for my family has shown me one very important thing: in your eyes and in God's, one child really does matter.

Sincerely,

Bijay

There's really no need to elaborate on the letter. It says it all.

After a forty-five-minute drive outside of Kathmandu, we found ourselves once again in a fairly remote area requiring a fifteen-minute trek to the project. We walked single file, exchanging hellos with the wonderful people of Nepal, passing stalls with meat lying on tables that had been there for days. Flies were everywhere; there were vegetable stalls, small kiosks with vendors selling different wares, and people just sitting in the street living life, a life that was simple yet hard. For all of that, they seemed pleased with who they were and what they had, which was nothing much, but to them it was everything, and that is all they needed. We, on the other hand, saw things differently. We saw people who were poor and living in places we couldn't imagine living in. We saw people smiling when we would have been crying. We saw children wearing no shoes as they played in dirty, torn clothes, laughing and having fun just like children in a developed country. We wondered how and why all who we saw were at peace with who they were and with what they had. My conclusion was that it was because they knew nothing else and were content to have just what they needed and nothing more. To be content with so little is a Gospel value, and when we are immersed in the affluence of the western world, it is a hard road, as Jesus put it, to find true spiritual treasure. We teach and counsel in all the countries to which we travel, and yet we never fail to be taught by those we serve.

The next project we went to was a school, a nice one with relatively new buildings, children in uniforms, and teachers who were well versed in their profession. It was a wonderful place to grow and learn. My assessment of the children was very positive. They were in good health, physically and emotionally. Their nutritional status was good, and they had a positive outlook on life and a good relationship with God. Our children there were thriving. They had a balanced meal every day, teachers who cared, a focus on God, and a school with a mission to teach them to learn and embrace life. At the end of the day, they sang for us, clapped in thanks for us being there, and high-fived us as they passed us on their way home.

We had climbed another few thousand feet on our trek to the summit of improved healthcare for the children. In turn, they had reached a summit where they could look out over the world and say, "Yes, this is mine, and I am healthy enough, knowledgeable enough, and spiritually filled to go out into this world and live a life that is full and not be hungry, dirty, and sick."

For me, the last day of clinics was the hardest since we saw several children for whom we could do nothing. The very last patient of the day was brought to me, an eighteen-month-old girl with a large head. She hadn't started walking yet and was carried by her mother, who wanted to know why her child was behind in her development. When she'd taken her daughter for immunizations a few months earlier, a physician had told her that all was well. Her daughter clearly had a condition called hydrocephalus (water on the brain), and without surgery she would soon die. As a critical care physician, sharing bad news is something that I do frequently. But sharing unwanted news through an interpreter with a mother who for the first time was hearing that her daughter would need surgery in order to avoid death was that much harder. In the mother's words, the father was a drunkard. He was there as well and also looked shocked as I related to them the seriousness of the situation. Why, then, didn't we just give them a handful of money and send them to a hospital to get the surgery. There would have been a happy ending, and everyone could have lived a richer and happier life.

But it wasn't that simple. With hydrocephalus, there's a need for follow-up care and rehab. There is also a high rate of infection in such cases, and an even higher chance that a shunt used to control the hydrocephalus—a drainage tube with a valve to relieve pressure on the brain—would require modifications or replacement. All this represents enormous financial costs. The family lived far from Kathmandu and had no money for transportation for frequent visits to the hospital. When I think of our sponsored children, we have a way to at least address issues like this one. We have in place a medical referral process that allows us to look at every case, see if we can contribute financially, and then assess whether or not we can help within certain limits. Like so many, this little girl wasn't sponsored.

A couple of days earlier, a mother and her two daughters had come to the clinic. Their father had passed away a few months back, and they were emotionally drained. We were fortunate to have a child psychologist (Dr. John) with us, who did a wonderful job counseling them while Pastor Michael did a great job with the spiritual side. Our team was made up of many people, each with gifts and talents that God had given them, and together we served. We reached the summit, but I wasn't ready to raise the flag just yet. We needed to go back and make the climb again—and maybe again after that—to reach our goal of sustainability.

Jesus took three disciples one day—Peter, James, and John—and climbed a mountain, where his face and clothes were suddenly bathed in a brilliant white light. The event is called The Transfiguration. Jesus began to talk to Moses and Elijah, who suddenly appeared on the mountain as a cloud covered all those present. Peter said, "Lord, it is wonderful for us to be here; if you wish, I will make three tents, one for you, one for Moses and one for Elijah" (Matthew 17:4/JB). Quickly, however, the cloud vanished, along with Moses and Elijah, leaving Jesus and His disciples alone again, everything having returned to normal.

I think most people can relate to Peter's statement: Lord, it is good to be here. Peak experiences are mysterious and awe-inspiring, just as when I looked at Everest and the climbers who were going to conquer the mountain. When we operate at our best and with maximum efficiency, we feel more alive and energized. On our Medical Mercy trips, we also feel more aware of His glowing presence as we carry out His will. There's something about reaching a goal, or even just the experience of the climb, that sharpens our focus, helping us to see beyond our normal everyday experience, as was the case with Peter, James, and John. Short of becoming permanent missionaries, however, the day comes when it's over and we must descend from our encounters with His people and return to our homes and the workaday world.

And yet I never really forget what the summit looked like. Many years later, Peter recalled his experience on the mountain in his epistle (2 Peter 1: 15-18), in which he says that he saw Christ's majesty on the mountain with his own eyes, a time when God said, "This is my Son, the Beloved; he enjoys my favor" (2 Peter: 17/JB). We are meant to live in the everyday world, but all of our encounters with God are transformative. When I see the forgotten children, I am changed. When I see them, I am standing in God's radiant light. And I never forget either—neither the children nor the peak experience of serving. We cannot live on the summit indefinitely, but we are called to use our time in the brightness of His love, even on the gray days when we must use memory to recall it, to be ministers of His grace.

Whether I am in Phoenix or Nepal, I know to whom I

belong to. I would climb again in the years ahead, but whether I stand on a mountain or plain, I stand with Him. I had asked my team why they did what they did. They gave me their answers as I watched them serve the children regardless of whether they were sponsored or not. And they answered as I saw them pray for our patients each day as we climbed to the summit together. They did it for Him. To paraphrase Peter, it was good for all of us to be there.

Chapter Thirty-one

Servants

I am often asked how we choose the countries we go to. It's really not that complex. We go where we think the greatest need is for the children at that point in time, always informed by the Holy Spirit, of course. In October 2013, we were led to take our third trip to India, but to a different location. South, on the very tip of India, is an area called Kerala. It's nothing more than a sliver of land on the Malabar Coast bordering the Arabian Sea. We had several projects there, with many children who were in need of medical care and nutritional assessments.

I remembered India well. The children there had an aura of the unkempt, many with bags under their eyes, pouchy faces—faces that, more often than not, were sunken and void of all emotion—and hair coated with dirt. I recalled the times we were faced with making critical decisions as to whether or not we could help a child there. Most of the time we did, and it was that "most of the time" that stayed with me. As noted earlier, sometimes we can't help children because there are no medical facilities available that can offer the needed medical interventions if a referral is warranted. Other times, parents don't see the need to pursue medical treatment, believing in obscure spiritual healings that are contrary to the evidence that there needs to be a partnership between medicine and religion.

It's then that I realize that such critical moments arrive with astonishing suddenness and then are gone, without us being able to do anything about them.

Accordingly, I have come to realize that the decisions of our past are the architects of our present. I try to make the right decisions for my patients, but there are times when I operate in a moral gray area. How far do I go with limited resources while trying to have realistic expectations? It's the age-old battle between mind and heart, which seldom want the same thing. In covenant medicine, there is a clear point at which I need to step back and let natural processes of age or disease run their sad but unavoidable course, but that's not the same as dealing with patients for whom much could be done given different financial or geographical situations. Frequently it comes down to a judgment call, and all I can do is pray that I make the right one.

Whatever the case, I try in every situation to offer comfort by validating patients, affirming who they are as people. For me, each day that I'm with them is the "beginning of forever" in the sense that I want patients to remember that, even though we are with them for just a short time, we have affirmed that the power of the human spirit and faith can endure any challenge, no matter how daunting. In a less than perfect world, it's all we can offer those who can't or won't take the extra step, but it's a powerful interaction with those we see nonetheless.

Every now and then we have a day that we want to remember always—or possibly forget—a day that is so out of the ordinary, so different from all the rest that it strikes a chord in our hearts and minds and plays a tune that makes us smile or gives us pause. October 7th was one of those days.

Not knowing what to expect, we drove two hours to a

remote province where we walked down a dirt road to a hidden school haven, the children waiting. All were in uniform, with white shirts, pants, skirts, and blue ties for both boys and girls. This was quite unexpected. Where were the poor and the isolated? Where were the malnourished and the weak? Where were the sick? They were there, but hidden behind smiles and a sense of community in a school that offered an education and an opportunity to pursue a better life than the one the children were born into. Behind the uniforms and the smiles, however, were severe effects of malnutrition that resulted in stunting. Children looked years younger than they really were. I saw a nine-year-old who was the size of a six year old, and a twelve year old who looked to be seven. The stunting would produce long-term effects. Girls would deliver prematurely once they became women and got pregnant, and boys would grow up with weakened physiques, limiting them to vocations that would not necessarily give them an opportunity to achieve their greatest potential. They looked healthy on the outside, but were compromised for life due to malnutrition before the age of five. This was the tragedy behind the veil of presumed health.

We nevertheless left the school feeling like we had impacted lives. We ran through all of our usual protocols, making sure that the children knew they were treasured and cared for. It was a day of sadness behind our smiles, knowing that the children were going to suffer the effects of stunting for the rest of their lives, but it was also a day of happiness because we left something of our love and encouragement behind. It was indeed a day so out of the ordinary that it made us both smile and reflect. It was bittersweet, but what a wonderful day all the same.

For whatever reason, life comes at us from unexpected directions at times. That is not to say that all is bad, but simply to suggest that there are times when we expect certain things to go one way, but they veer far from the path we expect them to take. I expected to travel on a bumpy road to a project with significantly impoverished children who longed for a decent life. That's not what happened on day two in India. With good intentions, we traveled to our site, saw 185 children, identified many in need of advanced care, and participated in the feeding program, observing them eat their daily meal provided by One Child Matters. They were more nutritionally on target for their age compared to the children the day before, the ones who didn't have access to daily meals. Here was where expectations turned a little to the north—to the positive side. I expected to see children who were sicker, more malnourished, and more impoverished since we were in a locale much poorer than where we were on day one. While the children were, in fact, sicker and more impoverished, they were relatively well-nourished and well-adjusted despite the conditions they lived in. They were happy, content, and interactive. The project the children came from embraced a holistic approach in giving the children what they needed and deserved in order for them to experience life to their fullest potential. It was because of the dedication of the teachers, project leaders, pastors, and the local One Child Matters leadership that the children were moving in the direction of personhood and worth. This was astonishing confirmation of the power of love and the spirit of giving. A caring attitude trumped even disease and counterbalanced unfavorable living conditions. The dedication of the teachers and staff was literally bolstering the mental health of the children, keeping them away from depression, which is a gateway to many serious illnesses. Jesus cast out many demons from people when He walked the earth, but while there were no exorcisms going on in India, I could see that the leadership was keeping these little ones spiritually safe.

I also saw a child on the second day who was born with a significant discrepancy in leg length. He'd had surgery to correct his gait, the operation financially supported through the One Child Matters' Children's Crisis Fund. The boy walked with a limp now but was self-confident and played with the other children as if he were no different. It's things like this that make what we do worthwhile: giving a child a chance to be a child.

Five hours from where we were based, we traveled winding roads the following day, roads so narrow that only one bus could move in any direction. The terrain was mountainous, with monkeys, elephants, and rubber trees around us, far from the strip malls and skyscrapers that were part of our lives back home. We didn't return to our base until the end of the week, seeing children who had little if anything but wanted for nothing. It was a welcome pattern that was starting to emerge. They were happy with what they had, needing only meals and love.

These were the children who awaited us. Each had his or her own personality, unique smile, and a personal story that they were eager to share with us. They were happy despite all they faced and gave us hope that they would be okay. The project teachers, the principal, and the pastor were clearly engaged with these children and cared deeply about them. When we are this far from what we know as comfortable or familiar, we never cease to be amazed at the resilience of the children who live in an environment that would be totally alien to us. When there are people who "care enough to care," people can endure and even thrive in harsh conditions.

The team worked flawlessly at our next clinic. After the infectious enthusiasm of the children the previous day, nothing could slow us down. Everyone made the most of their individual talents and served the children. We still had to travel to two more clinics, and I waited to see where the road would take us, with no expectation of what we would see in the children. It was always nice to come upon smiling, happy faces of children who weren't as bad off as we expected them to be, but every place was different. Following His direction was what counted.

We'd seen over 1,100 children in four days, with one more day to go. It's never about the numbers, although we are always intrigued by the "number seen." It gives us a sense of accomplishment, a sense of completion. But that's just the big picture. We never forget the details.

She was eight but was the size of a five year old. She was chronically ill, had a persistent cough, pneumonia, no appetite, and demonstrated a lack of enthusiasm for life. She'd had no breakfast that morning, and there was no food in her house. According to the child, her parents had been quarreling. The mother was sick, and the father was rarely home. She was a sponsored child, and because of that she was one of the lucky ones. She got a noontime meal Monday through Friday because of the association One Child Matters had with the school that she attended. I gave her medications, put her into our follow-up system, and the local One Child Matters staff would follow her progress closely and send me a report after two weeks as to how she was doing. We did a full nutritional assessment on her, and she was to be assessed every six months after that. Without these measures, she would have passed away slowly—and alone. Hopefully, she would do well, grow, and be able to live a fulfilling life.

The number of patients seen is important, but the total number we treat at any clinic anywhere in the world is made up of individuals like this little girl. She didn't have an optimal home situation by any means, but with One Child Matters, she had people who cared about her. She had a chance.

After five days of clinics, two of which were half-days due to travel, we finished serving the 1,414 children that came to see us. The team was incredible. They worked tirelessly, without complaints and giving all they had. The theme for the week was "Who are you trying to please," based Galatians 1:10, the full text of which reads, "Am I now trying to win the approval of human beings, or of God? Or am I trying to please people? If I were still trying to please people, I would not be a servant of Christ" (NIV). I shared with the team that there are times when we are self-pleasing, people-pleasing, and God-pleasing, the latter not always occurring as frequently as it should. Unfortunately, we can slip into a mode of pleasing ourselves or others, especially when times are tough on these trips and we can't live up to our expectations. Maybe that's when we start looking at the number of people served and pat ourselves on the back, congratulating ourselves for doing what few others attempt. We can then call ourselves humanitarians and say that at least we're doing more than most. These things might be true, and there's nothing wrong in being proud of our accomplishments—that's simply part of good self-esteem—but at the end of the day we must remember that we're not secular humanists. We must always remain aware that we're servants of the one who created the forgotten children. Our missions are rooted in prayer and humility, and without God in the equation, I have no doubt in my own mind that the results at the end of our five-day clinics would be drastically different.

I am confident that the team felt the same way after we discussed the week and what had happened to both the children and us. Prayer, both silent and communal, was abundant the entire time we were there. It was time to go back to our crazy lives, but the children were better off than when we'd arrived, and we gave and received much hope as we moved through the week. We had been God-pleasers. We'd been servants, and for that we were all thankful.

Chapter Thirty-two
It Is What It Is

We journeyed back to Haiti yet again. After an earthquake and cholera epidemic, the country was still under a great deal of hardship and continued to need help despite the strides we'd made. We were scheduled to travel to twelve projects in five and a half days, seeing our children and patients in the community at large. The times would be tough, the roads rough, and the weather hot and humid. There was going to be little time for rest, but we would never want it any other way. Our medical ministry is to serve and to endure. Because of conditions in Haiti, we knew we'd see children and adults who were close to the end of their lives. It is great when we can produce happy outcomes, but there are numerous instances when we see the endgame in the battles against poverty and disease. But we are called to help any and everyone in any way we can, not simply a chosen few or the easy cases. As servants, we take what comes our way.

It was January 5, 2014. It snowed, and then it snowed some more, so much so that what should have been an eight-hour trip from Phoenix to the Dominican Republic took forty hours. Our team of twenty-seven was scattered, from Atlanta to Dulles to JFK to Miami. When everyone finally arrived, we had a three-hour drive to the border to cross into Haiti. It took two hours to negotiate the protocols of two different countries, but we made it across despite the bureaucracy. At the first project of our first clinic, the team came together, each member knowing where to go and what to do. There's an old saying in Hollywood when shooting a movie: "Don't lose the light!" We saw a bunch of children in the two hours we had left before night settled on us. We'd gotten our feet wet for the rest of the week.

The subject of expectation was on my mind the first day. I saw an eight-year-old girl who was the size of a five year old. She was stunted. I was struck by the persistence of a country still torn from decades of unrest, a cholera epidemic on the verge of reappearing, and an infrastructure literally broken from the earthquake a few years earlier. As for expectations, there were none beyond my trusting that God would be present with His people. Beyond that, I'd learned not to have any. That's not to say that I didn't maintain hope, for I'd seen the miracle of sustainability in follow-up visits to many countries. What was on my mind, however, had more to do with what the people themselves expected and what made them satisfied. In countries that were underprivileged and impoverished, the mindset was "It is what it is." But this isn't necessarily a fatalistic outlook. It can also reflect contentment and gratitude. Results are dictated by those who live in the regions we visit, and my spiritual journey was still teaching me that I had to adjust my own expectations to match those of the people I served.

Making a child healthier, receiving a smile, and knowing that her chance for living a life with potential is its own reward. But if that outcome governs *all* of my expectations, what was I to do with the remorse I felt when someone couldn't be helped—couldn't live a long life filled with achievements? I was again confronted by the plain truth that I couldn't make my life in Phoenix—or a life in any developed, technological country—the yardstick by which success was measured. People's happiness is measured by the cultural norms they are exposed to day in and day out, and the spiritual reality was that their expectations didn't always match mine or my team's. Jesus said that what was born of the flesh was flesh, but what was born of the Spirit was spirit, and a soul blessed by God will look at things in a totally different way—and usually a much simpler one.

One day Jesus saw Jews putting money into the Temple treasury (Mark 12: 41-44). Rich men put in large sums, while a poor widow put in two pennies. Jesus remarked that she'd put in more than anyone else. Why? Because measurements of happiness, accomplishment—even fulfilling one's duty, as with the widow—involve different standards of measurement, different expectations. What others expect, and what God Himself expects, is not always what we have in mind for a situation. I was learning to let go of expectations and allow God to determine what was right and best.

Sometimes I marvel at the end of the day at how many things that have been accomplished.

Using dirt roads blocked by pigs at several junctures, we traveled to two separate clinics in two different communities, both two hours from our hotel. We left at seven in the morning and returned to the hotel at eight that night. I recalled how Jesus walked on the water one night to find His disciples far out on the lake, the boat battling a headwind. When he neared their boat, the storm suddenly abated and the disciples looked about and saw that they had inexplicably arrived at their destination on the other side of the lake (John 6:16-21). I'm not quite sure how we saw 300 children at two separate and distant locations, but we did.

At one location we were cramped in a room, seeing children and conducting the pharmacy. We spotted a few serious illnesses and prevented one child from going blind due to a serious eye infection. It was a great feeling to know that we prevented someone from blindness, but by the same token it was sobering to think that blindness can be prevented so easily with some eye drops or antibiotics. While not every disease can be successfully treated, the resources are there to cure quite a few. What is lacking is the resolve in developed countries to eradicate disease and hunger, and that resolve can only be found by developing compassion and awareness.

As for the team, it caught that fever of caring and compassion as it always does when it sees lines of people waiting for a chance to better their lives and be free of pain and illness. It's as if our spirits respond by saying, "Yes! We're here! You've come to the right place." It was a long day, but there were smiles all around when we'd finished.

So we sometimes look around and say to ourselves "How can they live like this?" Those we serve, however, say, "We'd like it to be better, but it is what it is. We trust in God, and He is good." At least that is what a kind old crippled Haitian man said when he came up to me when I stepped out into their world to take pictures. I think he had it exactly right. God is good.

"Why are you so sad?" Dr. Jerry asked the child in front of him.

"Because I'm hungry" the young boy answered.

There's not much one can say after that, and it was one of those moments when one wished the question had never been asked. And yet it *had* to asked, for that was why we were there. But there was a hard truth in the stark simplicity of the exchange. One can view the third world and analyze its problems in endless ways, citing politics, economics, geography, lack of education, gangs, drugs, and a variety of other factors, but sometimes a simpler explanation lies beneath all of the other reasons. In this case, hunger caused sadness.

In developed countries, people experience a pain or a symptom and make a doctor's appointment. "So tell me why you're here today?" the physician asks his patient. The answer is usually straightforward. "I have stiffness in my knee. I have a sore throat. I'm not seeing as well as I used to." Perhaps we would stop trying to solve the problems of the third world with academic and philosophical theories as to why people can't (or should be able to) pull themselves up by their bootstraps if we focused on their simple needs. They hurt. They're born into situations over which they have no control. And yes—they're hungry.

And here is another bit of simplicity. It is part of the ministry of One Child Matters to feed children as best we can. They were given spaghetti with tomato sauce, a hardboiled egg, and a banana. It wasn't a meal fit for a king, but it was probably the best meal they'd have until they come back to the project for more. Good food. Nutritious food. And it was better than nothing.

Simplicity. Blindness is prevented with common medication. Hunger is relieved by a basic but nutritious meal. People are satisfied if they can see or eat a spaghetti dinner. That's their expectation for a good and happy life. Perhaps it should be that simple for everyone. We get upset if we can't buy a summer home or park a luxurious camper in our driveway. We want bigger flatscreen TVs and faster computers. Some kids just want to eat.

Jesus thanked His Father for revealing the kingdom, not to the learned and clever, but to mere children, meaning people without pretension or great expectations of wealth—or any expectations at all except to have their basic needs met. It was they who could appreciate His message of love and simplicity. Cripples walked again. The deaf could hear. That was enough for them, and they were grateful.

Sometimes it's hard to articulate the right thing to say—what's really on our minds and what's important. It was another day, with more children, different village communities, but the same basic scenario. But what was behind our purpose, mission, and priorities? From the Haitians I'd learned that their purpose was to stay alive. Their mission was to find where their next meal was coming from. Their priority was to fend for themselves as best they could in order to fulfill their purpose, completing a vicious circle. But the children we cared for were learning differently what these three categories meant. They were learning to purposely live a life with Christ, to serve others as their mission in life, and to make God their first priority. Even though they lived in squalor and poverty, they saw beyond their "have not" status and relished the "have" of a life filled with grace and love, a life lived in a community of dedicated servants. Their expectation was "It is what it is," only for them the "is" was living with and serving God, and that made them happier than many of the wealthiest people on the planet.

Day five brought us a two-hour drive on paths that only aspired to be roads. Climbing through the chain of mountains outside of Cap-Haitien, we saw a distant part of Haiti that was a mere speck on the side of the island, one that was far from the civilization on the east side called the Dominican Republic. The road twisted and yielded little in the way of comfort. We traveled slowly if only to prevent damage to our bodies and the van. We wouldn't be of any use to our patients if we couldn't complete the drive or arrive in decent enough shape to do our jobs.

We were supposed to see children in three projects. We arrived at the first and quickly realized that it wasn't going to happen. Going to three projects would be too arduous and time-consuming considering the terrain. Children were brought to us from the projects, and we stayed there all day, with a fifteen-minute break for lunch before the constant stream of children resumed.

I saw him out of the corner of my eye. With him was a tall elderly lady, unkempt, frail, and barley able to walk. He came and sat in the chair in front of me, waiting to be examined as he looked at me with a stoic face. He was only three but acted years beyond his age. I guess stoicism does that to a person. After asking only a few questions, I figured out his plight. His parents had abandoned him, and his grandmother had taken him in—and so had One Child Matters. He was a sponsored child, cared for by a frail and elderly woman who, I thought, might not be alive the next day. He was like many others we cared for. I spent some time with him and treated his malnutrition and chronic pneumonia. He didn't smile, but when I put him in my lap, he cuddled close and showed a soft smile as he laid his head against my chest. For him, love had been hard to come by. His expectation? To be held and loved. It doesn't get any simpler than that.

Later, the sun was setting as we sat on the bus that crept along the road that wasn't a road, and for a moment there was a pause in the conversation centering on the experiences everyone was sharing from the day's clinic. It was at that moment that it all came together for me. An abandoned three-year-old child had been given a chance to be loved and cherished by those who embraced him in the One Child Matters project. He had a chance because he had clean water to drink, a toothbrush, a band aid for his cuts, a teacher who knew how to treat a burn, a place to wash his hands, and a medical program that would administer preventative health exams. As in the Gospel, he had his two cents, and for him it was a fortune.

There comes a time when we realize that things need to come to an end. We finished up our last day of clinic, having seen 1,400 children, building two permanent "tippy taps" (for hand washing) in each of the eleven projects we went to as well as providing additional water filtration systems. But why is it so important to point out that which we do in so many locations? The reason is because when the end of each mission comes, we look back and wonder if the road we traveled was straight or meandering, and if we really arrived at our destination. For me, the answer was there on the last morning.

I was asked to look at an eleven-year-old girl who'd had surgery several years earlier to remove a superficial mass on her neck. She was left with nerve damage to her arm and an accumulation of lymph that caused her arm to swell to twice its normal size. She had a chest X-ray taken a while back when her mother took her to see a doctor after many years of wondering why her daughter's arm looked the way it did after surgery. The chest X-ray showed two masses in her chest. No one bothered to tell the mother what the findings were at the time the X-rays were taken, nor did the doctor who did the original surgery tell the mother what the mass was that he had removed. Those who took an oath to heal and care had abandoned the mother and the child. This time that didn't happen. Working with local doctors, I examined the child, came up with a plan on what tests were needed, what the next step in the care should be, sat with the mother and explained to her in detail what was going on, and promised to always be there for them. The expectation was simple: to recognize those who come to us for help as persons worthy of dignity no matter what their circumstances were. I believe we did that.

I have already alluded to the parable of the master who gave his servants talents in his absence so that they might carry out his business. To the servants who multiplied their talents, the master said, "Well done, good and faithful servant." We didn't give up on the eleven-year-old girl. We'd done our master's bidding, and I was sure, therefore, that the road we'd traveled had indeed been true.

And there was that word again: servant. When we remember that's what we are—servants—the road stays straight. That's also the expectation God has for us—to serve. It's the only expectation that we need to worry about.

Chapter Thirty-three

Obstacles

Overcoming obstacles would be the theme for the upcoming trip to Kenya in May of 2014. So why the theme? We're all faced with obstacles that need to be overcome. Sometimes we can't get over the hurdle and must seek another way to get where we want to go. The week before we were scheduled to leave, I realized that there was indeed an obstacle that we would face, and I prayed that we were up to the task. I'd been on clinical service in the pediatric critical care unit in Phoenix and had been taking care of children who were on the edge of life. They had traumatic brain injuries, cancer, life-threatening infections, and many more illnesses. One child in particular caught my attention as I speculated how we would deal with similar situations if we came across them in Kenya. The little boy had a devastating kidney disease requiring that both his kidneys be removed, necessitating that he live on dialysis for several years. He was on the transplant list for a kidney, but the list is always long, and kidneys are hard to come by. As a last resort, his mother asked if she could be tested to see if her kidney would be compatible. One would think that since she was his mother, the kidney would certainly be a match, but the compatibility factors a doctor has to consider are numerous, and the chances of a mother having a compatible kidney for her son were marginal at best. Luckily, her kidney matched. The little boy received his mother's right kidney and was on his way to living a normal life again, gifted by his mother, with the surgery done in a healthcare system that had the technology and services to make the miracle happen. So this was the obstacle: could this ever happen in Kenya, and what would we do if we came up against something like this while we were there? Sustainable care has limits. Dialysis in Kenya is hard to come by, and kidney transplants are rare. We would be treating a population that was isolated from advanced services of all kinds, if we could even call the services available there "advanced." The scenario of a Kenyan child who needed a kidney, with a mother who would gladly donate her own, would not play out the same way it had in Phoenix. I hoped that I wouldn't be faced with anything of this nature, but it can and does happen all the same. There was no way of knowing for sure, but our teams were routinely faced with many obstacles as we served those who came to us, one being the inability to deliver much-needed medical care because of a lack of resources through no fault of our own.

And so the question hung in my mind in the days leading up to the trip: what exactly would we do? We would, of course, pray. Sometimes miracles happen, even big ones, but as I already said, it's a question of adjusting expectations to fit the reality of the regions we visit. The only thing to do is to place a situation in His hands and hope for the best.

Darkness fell on the day we arrived, and then it got darker still. From the edge of night to the beginning of dawn, we were flying 37,000 feet above the earth, traveling at 580 miles per hour. I feigned sleep, but I was only fooling myself. There were too many things on my mind—too many thoughts, too many "what ifs." They swirled around the tired neurons in my brain that longed for rest. They weren't full-blown worries, but simply thoughts of anticipation of what we would be up against. There was one thing that gnawed at me, however, and that was the silent prayer we would maintain in public. These are troubled times, when the open declaration of a faith is targeted in countries that are self-righteous in their *own* faith, leaving little, if any, room for others to express their personal belief in God. We wouldn't force the issue or cause conflict, but the self-imposed silence would be different for us this time around.

I was reminded of an event that had occurred recently. At a university, the dictum was that graduation speakers, including the student valedictorian, could not reference God in their speeches. When a particular student valedictorian approached the podium to give his speech, he sneezed, and as planned, the whole graduating class yelled out "God bless you!" I shared this with the team to see how we could use it as an example of a not-so-subtle declaration of faith. It was worth a shot.

It would all start the next day on ravaged roads leading to an isolated project. When the sun touched the horizon in the morning, yielding a burst of orange light, we would head out and begin to see those waiting for us.

All dirt roads. It was slow going, and the sky opened up, rain pouring down as we sought shelter in a mud building with a tin roof. The noise of the rain beating down on the tin drowned out all the breath and heart sounds we were trying to listen to as we examined the children, so right off the bat we had an obstacle, but we remained patient and did our best. A few children with serious diseases were identified and referred to local hospitals, but malnutrition was the diagnosis of the day.

The girl was ten years old and complained of fatigue. She had a history of a high fever, weakness, and shortness of breath. Her heart was pounding so hard that I could see her chest heave with each beat. She clearly had an enlarged heart and congestive heart failure, probably stemming from rheumatic heart disease. She received intervention and care during the week, and we left for the hotel at six in the evening. I'd been right about obstacles. They were coming at us pretty fast.

More rain fell the next day—a lot of it—and a dirt road washed out. Three vans carrying the U.S. team made it to the clinic site in two hours, but the bus carrying the meds and the healthcare workers slid off the road, causing a big delay. After several hours, everyone arrived and the clinic started. Obstacles.

Not all obstacles were attributable to the weather, however. The boy was nine. There had been nothing abnormal about his health until he turned one and half years old, when he developed a high temperature and what sounded like meningitis. This wasn't good news for a child in the African bush. He had survived, but with significant deficits, both mental and physical. He experienced three to five seizures a month even on medication. He was one of our sponsored children, and after I examined him, we worked on getting him to a school for special needs. I'm committed to caring for all children and giving them the best hope for achieving their God-given potential. They deserve no less.

Traveling for two hours over bumpy and treacherous roads in unpredictable weather was all worth it once the voices of the children were heard. As the convoy approached the project of the day, we heard songs of joy and happiness from hundreds of children wanting to greet us. It was clear that much effort was put into their greeting, which showed their level of gratitude. Hundreds of hands were extended in welcome. They probably didn't know quite what to expect, other than that U.S. doctors were going to try to make them healthier, but their level of trust was astounding.

Throughout a day of examining and poking, they maintained this degree of trust. A little boy had jiggers (parasitic fleas) boring holes into his feet. Even though he was unsure what was happening while his painful sores were cleaned and scrubbed, he remained composed, trusting that we were there to help. He cried when he left the clinic, but he appeared a few hours later, playing soccer on his newly healed feet while giving us high fives with a big smile on his face. It showed us the resilience of the mind, body, and spirit in the presence of genuine love and caring. Not all results are manifested so quickly, but it was a reminder that we bring the "good news" of the Gospel: change is possible.

The second patient was a young woman who complained of stomach pain. She told us of her habit of breaking off pieces of the mud walls of her house and how she consumed them. Her gums and conjunctiva were white. Her behavior indicated that she suffered from pica, a psychological disorder marked by eating nonorganic substances such as clay, dirt, paint, and other materials that can be harmful to the body. It was almost a "textbook illness" since the condition is rarely seen in most countries. We wondered if she understood her condition. Did she think she was crazy? Whatever the case, her level of comfort with her examiners was obvious, demonstrating the physician-patient relationship at its best.

It had been a successful day. The enthusiasm with which

we were greeted continued throughout the clinic. The boy with jiggers, the woman with pica, and dozens more like them indicated that they trusted us and were grateful for the care they received. This wasn't always the case—some patients left a clinic with sadness, suspicion, or outright disappointment—but it was always good when we could see tangible results and connect with patients whose gratitude was demonstrable.

He was quiet and withdrawn, unwilling to look me in the eye. Upon examination, I saw massive lymph nodes, which indicated that he had a serious chronic illness. I had a hunch as to what it might be, but how could I approach it delicately and with compassion? *What* we see is not necessarily *who* we see. His withdrawal was not a reflection of who he was. He was an abandoned child, ill and wanting confirmation of his worth. We put a hand on his shoulder, looked him in the eye, and made him feel loved. From these simple gestures, he knew that we would try to help him get well.

We treated a severe leg burn on a two year old, and several children were sent to the hospital for emergency medical care. But just because we were there for the children didn't mean we neglected adults who came to us with significant problems. A forty-year-old mother came to us complaining of a "wound in her womb." Translators were unable to help us sort out what she was attempting to describe, but she'd had eleven children, two of whom had died, one right after birth and another at the age of six from what sounded like meningitis. She'd also had severe complications during her pregnancies and deliveries. We knew what to do and, more importantly, where to send her for the fifteen-minute operation that would change her life and end the wound in her womb.

We heard many stories of chronic illnesses in children who simply needed guidance. The beauty in this was that the healthcare workers—the ones who identified these children—knew where to send them and needed only our assurance that they were, in fact, right in their assessments.

So what's it like to go on a medical mission trip? Thinking ahead and anticipating what one wants to accomplish is likely to leave a person with regret and frustration when expectations aren't met. Over the years I have found that it's best to have an open mind. That is what worked best on the trip to Kenya. Things changed, plans were made anew, and some were canceled, but things still fell into place (which I always suspect is God's doing). It comes back to obstacles, because most of the time they're going to be encountered even though some days surprise us and everything flows smoothly, with the protocols and clinic tracks operating with clockwork precision.

Jesus spoke of obstacles when he said that if believers had faith the size of a mustard seed, they could move mountains. Nothing would be impossible. These are encouraging words, and it's certainly important to stay grounded in faith. We nevertheless have to acknowledge that anything we do is part of a larger scheme, a thread woven into a complex tapestry, and the ultimate vision of what it's supposed to look like isn't something we, as fallible humans, are privy to. I believe that faith has to be tempered with humility so that we always remember that, despite our plans and intentions, God has a plan for every patient and clinic that we visit. Jesus said, "Ask and you shall receive, seek and you will find, knock and the door shall be opened." These, too, are encouraging words, implying that all prayer is answered. I truly believe that. But maybe our prayers are answered in different ways than we expect them to be answered, and perhaps the result comes on a time schedule that doesn't mesh with ours. Many stories have been written about God's intervention in which a seemingly disappointing event was exactly what precipitated a miracle. Quite a few people have been delayed, caught in traffic, missed flights, lost jobs, and suffered all manner of setbacks, only to find that these annoyances worked for their good in the long run. The accounts are too numerous to list in which a delay saved someone from being caught in a building that exploded or boarding a flight that crashed—and so on. Do I believe that mountains are moved? Yes, although I can't always explain the how, when, where, or why. And sometimes I simply believe that they'll be moved even if I don't see it happen. Or perhaps a different mountain altogether is moved than the one I was looking to see vanish.

So what am I getting at? Faith is a hard road to travel because one must walk a fine line between believing that God is at work versus surrendering a situation to Him. On our mission trips, supplies and personnel sometimes show up out of the blue, and a patient for whom we hold out little hope is cured through a combination of prayer and medicine. Other times, God says no, as He did with Pastor. Still other patients are helped, but only to a certain extent. Others are too sick and there is little we can do for them except show our love. Where is the rhyme and reason? It's always with Him. Looking at seeming failure while retaining a mindset that God turns everything to the good is difficult because we have to walk blindly, content not to see the answer to a prayer, at least not as we might envision it.

One goes on a mission trip, therefore, with hope and love—and an acceptance that we will probably see things we can't figure out. This is what I mean by curtailing expectations. It's not that we don't expect to help people and be of service, but rather that we don't try to put God, along with every patient we see, into a category of completely successful outcomes.

Jesus said it very plainly: "Obstacles indeed there must be" (Matthew 18:7/JB). He didn't promise a smooth road, but it's a good road nonetheless, one that's straight and true. I don't know what lies ahead, but I wouldn't take any other road. At the end of the day, I can look with my mind's eye at some of the really tragic stories I've come across and unburden myself by acknowledging that I can't understand everything that happens.

Remember the god in a white coat I once was decades earlier? I'm glad he's gone. When we step off our pedestals and become servants, obstacles are a little easier to cope with.

Chapter Thirty-four
Do Not Be Afraid

Watching the orange glow of a rising sun touch the horizon, I took in all that was before me. Standing on the balcony of the Teo Hotel years ago on one of my very first trips to Cambodia, I smelled the odors and the fragrances—some nice, some not so nice—as I looked at the streets beginning to fill. The noise grew louder, families traveled to school and work, vendors pulled their carts, and beggars lined the street and the sidewalks, asking for alms. Smoke rose from a large funneled stack containing the ashes of those being cremated in the building below it and spoke of what was to come for all of us. All who come to life leave sooner or later, but I was there to ensure that those who came to see us would have a long and meaningful life.

That was many years ago, and since then Medical Mercy has made trips to fifteen countries. The next trip on our schedule was Cambodia in March of 2015. I am always amazed how a team comes together within a few short hours on the first day, giving of themselves and asking for nothing. That comes from the virtue of serving others while making our own concerns secondary.

But what exactly is serving others? It's sacrifice, as well as looking beyond the sadness, poverty, and helplessness of frail people who seek nothing more than a hand to hold. Lest you think these trips are merely a series of depressing moments, they're not. There are moments of smiles, gratitude, happiness, and a genuine covenant bond between us and our patients, something I call the "care covenant," a commitment to care regardless of the situation.

One would think that after twenty hours of flying, we would reach out to a bed and try to rest before hundreds of patients showed up at the clinic, but this wasn't the case. Excitement trumped exhaustion, and the mind moved our bodies gracefully but slowly as we anticipated all that we were going to see and do over the next few days.

A while back, an NGO was visiting a village and noticed that the women would get up early every morning and walk two hours to a river to get water for the day and then walk back. That was four hours of making sure that a valuable source of life was available for all those in the village. The NGO decided that a water well was needed, so they spent the next year and a great deal of money building a well in the village. Problem solved. But the villagers, although grateful, were not overly-joyous about the well. When asked why, they said that if they had been asked what their greatest need was, it would have been a school, as well as schoolbooks for the children. The women walking to get water had been a process that was readily accepted and had never been considered a burden. What was important was educating the children. The NGO had its eyes opened. It was further validation that we have to look at a village through the eyes of its inhabitants, not our own. What gives meaning to one life might be inconsequential to another.

When we arrived, we learned that mosquito nets treated with a chemical repellent were handed out by the hundreds to villagers who lived on coastal waters. Malaria was rampant, and the NGO's focus and expectation was to decrease the malaria rate. After a few months, the NGO heard that there was an increase in an unknown illness that was affecting the villagers, one even worse than malaria, so they retraced their steps and realized their mistake. The villagers were primarily fishermen, and because fishing nets were expensive and scarce, the mosquito nets treated with the chemical repellent were being used to catch fish. The result was that villagers were eating contaminated fish, and over a period of time the toxic repellant had accumulated in the villagers to produce illness. It wasn't anything that could have been predicted and was another example of how we can't plan for all contingencies. How could one foresee that a village would value schoolbooks over a close source of potable water? How could one anticipate that villagers were sick because they were using poisoned fishing nets to earn a living?

We can bring medical equipment and unload stethoscopes and blood pressure cuffs when we arrive at a village, but it's more important to unload preconceived notions about how things will work. Perhaps these moments are a way of reminding us that "the other" is more important than the self. What *we* do and how *we* live is not how people in other parts of the world act and live. I think this is a prerequisite for any kind of service to others: stepping back from the ego.

ᔕᗞ ᑕᘏ

As the warmth of the early morning sun broke through the waning darkness of the night, we drove 180 kilometers from Siem Reap to Battambang. Salaa Hope School was our first stop, and within thirty minutes we were up and running. The children all looked healthy and, in fact, they were. Salaa Hope was the school where we built our first medical clinic in 2004 and was staffed by Chhaiden, our country medical director. In 2005 I trained fifteen teachers to be healthcare workers, and Chhaiden showed a unique knack for the vocation. We sent him to medical school, and as a physician, he was responsible for the healthcare of the 3,000 One Child Matters children in Cambodia. Since 2004, we'd had in place a medical clinic, fifteen healthcare workers, and now a country medical director. It was true sustainable care and another answer to those who say we simply make hit and run visits, with things returning to the way they were in a relatively short time. When God wants to make His presence felt, there's no stopping Him.

In the afternoon we went to Prey Dach School, where there were a few hundred more children to see. There was no electricity, sweltering heat, and some minor technical problems with our new electronic medical records, all of which led to delays, but once we got going, we hit our stride.

So was there a story, a tale of an individual who was rescued from some terrible affliction? No, there were only smiles, laughs, and love from the children. It's always the little things that bring the biggest rewards. Despite the intense heat, I think we accomplished what we went there to do. Over many years, I've learned that, in the short term, the verification for this comes from the heart. As scripture says, what is born of the flesh is flesh, and what is born of the Spirit is spirit. I truly believe that the spirit of a man or woman is far more discerning than the eyes and ears.

Sometimes we can't hide from the truth, and the truth was that we didn't see many patients the next day. I could be a great wordsmith and write around the fact that we waited and waited for more patients to arrive, but it didn't happen. We sat around, getting to know each other, seeing only 100 patients. We ate lunch, went for a walk, visited a silk farm, and wondered what had happened. We were told that the children knew we were coming, but they were mostly adolescents and rather self-disciplined as to what they would or wouldn't do. Our theory was that since it was so hot, the teens were probably not keen on riding their bicycles in the heat and might come by around four of five in the afternoon.

What do you do when you sacrifice your time and travel 11,000 miles to do a medical mission trip and then wait for someone to show up? You question if it was a bust, a waste of time. If the truth be told, we all had this very thought. We sat around fanning ourselves and drinking liters of water and talking, but little did we know that a big change was on the way.

It had been a relatively restful time, needed and appreciated, but on the following day the clouds turned black, blocking out the sun. Torrential rain fell, drowning the country and all who lived in it. The rainy season was upon us. People looked around and continued to live life, thankful for the rain, undeterred by flooded streets, humidity, or dampness. They'd waited for it. It would last a few months, giving life to the dry arid land that Cambodia became in the dry season.

That is how it is in Cambodia, flipping from one season to the next. The next day we saw and lived in the dry season again, crawling along a shallow river of water to a lake where about 200 families lived on floating bamboo and wood houses, their lives governed by the ups and downs of the lake. In the rainy season the lake is swollen, with a water level thirty feet above the riverbed. Today, the floating village lay close to land both to the side and underneath them. There were about 300 children there in a school that was built by One Child Matters, so we set up clinic on the banks of the shallow lake as children came to us in small skiffs. We, too, had traveled several miles in small skiffs to get there. In the middle of a shallow lake in the boonies of Cambodia, working under tarps with a generator and a router, we saw a couple of hundred children and used our electronic medical record system—technology in a place barren of anything that would resemble comfort or modern trappings. The school had outhouses that emptied directly into the lake where the children swam. There was a cell phone tower a few hundred yards from the floating homes, with the school occupying a small patch of land in the lake, but they didn't have electricity or running water. The living conditions were mirrored by the health of the children, who were malnourished and had chronic infections. There was much to do and much to address. Even if we successfully treated the malnutrition and infections, swimming in the polluted water would theoretically override anything we could accomplish, but we had gained ground since we were last in Cambodia. Teaching the children about hygiene and bathroom protocols had made a difference. Yes, we saw some sick children, but they were better than what we saw several years ago. Sometimes it takes a lot of time, but we pressed on, unwilling to lose the ground we had previously gained.

The next morning I gave a talk on child abuse at one of the several clinical pearls I do each morning while we're on a medical mission trip. We talked about the presentation of symptoms, treatment, and protection of the child. By the same token, we were forced to talk about cultural differences when it came to parenting and what we ourselves consider child abuse in the West. Should we impose our cultural standards of child protection on other cultures, or should we try to understand the other side and look at what is considered acceptable discipline when a child is being hit with a stick? And what about the medical side? Coining is when a coin is rubbed hard on the skin, making significant red streaks over the back and the chest. Its purpose? To rid the child of fever and bad humors, and it was a common practice where we were. But what about something more disturbing, such as placing a burning ember on the skin in various patterns in order to (according to the local medicine man) rid the body of bad humors? This was performed on children who were held down and burned, and we saw such a child that day. When Cambodians working with us were asked about it, they shrugged their shoulders in general acknowledgement that it was a cultural norm. We struggled with the situation and wondered how we could teach the concept of caring, but without harming the child. The answer wasn't simple. The Cambodians didn't see it as harmful, but rather as a valid pathway to help cure a child of disease. For them it demonstrated a parent's love, no different than our own desire to protect children from illness. To us, however, the practice was incomprehensible. We shook our heads and hoped that some insight as to what constituted child abuse would cross cultural boundaries one day.

Hands on the shoulders of those in front of them, patients moved in a line through nutritional assessment and then waited to be seen by a medical provider. Each person had a different facial expression. Some smiled, while others were nervous and not sure what to expect. Some took in everything, and others looked like they had been through the entire process before. I remember one little boy in particular. He was shy, eyes downcast, hands twisting nervously, feet moving from side to side. I watched him as he was weighed and measured for height. He never looked up, but obeyed instructions and moved from one station to the next. One always questions coincidences, or at least I do. With fifteen medical examiners working while hundreds of children moved through the line in a manner that resembled orderly chaos, he was brought to me. Coincidence? I didn't think so. He sat down in front of me, eyes diverted. He ignored my smile even though my hand was on his as a form of gentle assurance that all would be well. Sitting back, I looked at him and stayed silent for a moment. I didn't have an interpreter, so I took a chance.

"Do you know who I am?" I asked in English.

He didn't reply.

"Do you know why you are here?"

He didn't look up. I thought it was probably silly of me to expect him to understand English and to respond, so I tried another approach.

"Can I hold your hand? Will you let me listen to your heart?"

He looked up, making eye contact as he reached out his hand. I took it, and we sat like that for a few moments, not saying anything. I simply held his hand and smiled, and he smiled back. I leaned in and put my stethoscope on his chest and heard his heart beating fast. As I continued to listen while holding his hand, his heart began to beat more slowly and his breathing became more regular.

I asked an interpreter sitting at another table to ask the little boy if he spoke English. When asked, he shook his head no, but he smiled at me and reached out for both of my hands and held them tightly. I held tightly, too, and then asked him if I could finish examining him. He said nothing, but let go of my hands. I finished the exam, and he looked at me and smiled the entire time.

When I was done, I filled out his form and gave him the plastic bag he would use to get his vitamins, tooth brush, a small gift, stickers, and an antibiotic I prescribed for an ear infection. He stood, started to walk away, and then stopped. He turned, looked at me, and smiled. I smiled back. I watched him for a long time as he made his way through the line to the rest of the stations. As he came to the last one, he turned around yet again and smiled at me one last time. I, of course, smiled back one last time. He was only five, but how did all this happen? Did he understand English? I'll never know, but I remembered what I'd told the team on many occasions: it's what we leave behind that's important. I'll never forget that five-year-old boy, and I hope he never forgets me. I have no way to figure out our brief transaction or dwell on the whys and the hows, but there was no need to. I had expected God's hand to touch those who came to see us, and that's exactly what happened: He gave that child a heart that understood me, a heart that miraculously opened up because he saw acceptance and love in my approach.

When children approached Jesus on numerous occasions, His disciples always tried to send them away, but Jesus rebuked them each time, saying, "Let the little children alone, and do not stop them coming to me; for it is to such as these that the kingdom of heaven belongs" (Matthew 19:14/JB). When the children had gathered around Him, He blessed them and touched them. Notice the two different approaches to the small and innocent. "Go away! Don't bother the master!" The other approach was, "Come here and be touched, loved, and blessed." One method pushes people away and closes down a person's mind and spirit. The other welcomes people and reaches out to them in love. But here's the point: holding someone's hand and smiling are simple acts. They cost nothing but are integral in covenant medicine, which advocates that first and foremost we become present to our patients.

When we conduct a clinic, we call children to us and welcome them with open arms. Given the harsh ways of the world and the rejection that so many of the forgotten children have experienced, is it any wonder that these little ones are often frightened and suspicious? No, but the first step is to do what Jesus did: affirm their importance and convey to them by whatever means possible the message used by God and His ministering angels in the New Testament: "Do not be afraid."

What did it all add up to? We'd seen toxic fishing nets, a village floating on a lake filled with human waste, and oppressive heat that kept teens inside, leaving us little to do but talk as opposed to engaging in our usually hectic schedule. A simple answer might be that every place—and everybody—is different, but maybe that line of reasoning is more simplistic than simple. The answer is too obvious. So what's happening at a deeper spiritual level?

Jesus said that the kingdom of God was like a dragnet cast into the sea that brings in a haul of all kinds (Matthew 13:47). Surely that's what my teams and I saw everywhere we went: a haul of all kinds. True, some things are constant in human nature, and the need for love and healthcare is uniform across the globe, but we also see an amazing diversity of situations, scenarios that can't be predicted. Our nets bring in the young and the old, the frightened and the trusting, the hopeful and the despondent. There are children in schools and children who are abandoned. There are patients who will get better, and there are patients who will die despite our best efforts. And yet God wishes to gather everyone, to bring them into His kingdom. In our many travels, we see firsthand just how wide and broad His net is, and we can see that He doesn't discriminate against anyone.

I see many things that break my heart and many things that I can't explain. But one thing I do know with utter certainty: His people are out there, and He wants them. Despite the many ills in the world, how can anyone not smile at the love that reaches out for us in every way imaginable? Perhaps we are all that five-year-old boy—a little suspicious and a little afraid—but we're all sitting on the lap of our heavenly Father.

Chapter Thirty-five

Good Samaritans

Father Time tapped me on the shoulder and asked, "Are you ready to go?"

I didn't reply.

"Are you ready to go?" he repeated, this time enunciating each word, each louder than the one preceding and with a pause in between them.

"No, I'm not," I softly said.

It was a foolish question that deserved no answer—or perhaps one that was at least honest. Who is ever ready for what we were about to do? Sure, we're ready with flight reservations, medications, clusters of clothes, and general "stuff" that we always need to pack, plus our music and reading material, but I, for one, was not mentally, emotionally, or spiritually ready. But how could that be after this many years? The answer is that it's hard to enter into a world so unlike my own, a world of severe poverty, sadness, hunger, illness, and want. We were going to India, a country of slums and waste, a mass of people who have little chance of finding any meaningful space of their own. But we continue to do it because, as servants, we are compelled to go by someone greater than ourselves. And so I prayed, as I do before each trip. For me, prayer prepares me for whatever is waiting out there. I find solace in the fact that there will be someone who will be in charge, someone who will carry the torch, someone who will lead the way. I just need to follow. So when my Father asked me a week later if I was ready, the answer was an unequivocal "yes." I had prayed, packed, paid the bills, prayed some more, given my last lectures, and did some clinical time in the PICU. I was ready!

We arrived after a thirty-six hour journey. You would think the trip there tedious, but while flying we are detached for many hours and miles—11,000 miles, in fact. Such solitude comes rarely these days in our busy world, and flying above the rim of the world for long durations gives us time to reflect, ponder, dream, and drift off without having to worry about the inevitable interruptions, requests, emails, texts, or banter that our lives are frequently burdened with. So I reflected and prepared my heart and mind for the six days of clinics that we would hold in remote projects and villages. Sometimes I need to climb to 38,000 feet and find some quiet time to remember that God puts us in places where we may not think we belong, but where we are needed all the same. I doubt that the original twelve apostles ever envisioned themselves traveling to Rome, Western Europe, Turkey, and even India after Jesus ascended into heaven, but that's where the Holy Spirit sent them. I wonder what kind of thoughts they entertained as they walked along those empty, ancient roads. I'm sure they prayed and reflected about what was ahead. I was in good company.

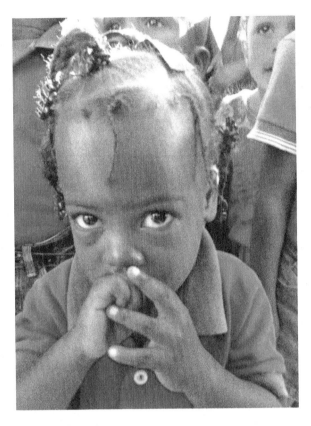

The boy walked over to me slowly, his eyes shifted to the side. Sitting, he placed his hands in his lap, sat forward, and looked everywhere but at me. He was twelve but was the size of a six year old. Stunted and malnourished, he was shy, introverted, and clearly uncomfortable. Taking his hand, I held it for a moment, saying nothing, and then I simply looked at him and smiled. He turned and looked at me, a faint smile appearing on his face, if only for a moment. I asked if I could take his picture so as to remember his smile, and he smiled just a little bit more, but his eyes said it all. His face was a combination of sadness and hope, but we connected. We had established a relationship of trust, that unspoken covenant and singular moment of understanding between two people without benefit of words.

Another boy shuffled over, displaying a look of wonder and uncertainty as to what this was all about. This four year old had a slightly cherubic face, although he had a no-nonsense character and an attitude that begged for an invitation to engage, but only on his terms. And that's what I did. I took his hand and held it for a moment. He quickly withdrew his hand and held it close in his lap. He wanted no part of the relationship I was trying hard to establish, so I tried again, but there was no chance of winning him over. He was healthy, well nourished, and sure of himself.

I wondered at how different and yet how much the same the two boys were. Both were born into the same community, had the same exposure to hardships, and the same opportunities given to them, although these were certainly limited. One was stunted, malnourished, and destined for a life of poor health and poverty. The other was a little fat, with an attitude of "I can do anything," destined for a life that would lead him to a much better place than the first boy. It was interesting to consider how relationships often exist between those who are fragile and those who are willing to brave the world. They were the same, and yet they weren't. But even more interesting was the fact that God loved each boy for who he was. Remember that dragnet I spoke of in the last chapter? It was right before me, and I marveled at the diversity of life on earth and how God, its author, honors all of it. It was a bit humbling in light of the fact that most of us are so filled with prejudices of one kind or another, even if they are small or unconscious. It was another reminder for the need to strive for agape, that unconditional love and acceptance of those who may be quite different from us—and each other.

It seems that we are sometimes given tasks that we just can't put our arms around. We're given shoes that don't quite fit, but we do the tasks anyway, and if we have no other shoes, then we squeeze into those given to us.

I saw a boy of twelve, his head held high. He had no lack of confidence, and a character that practically guaranteed that he was capable of doing anything. I looked at his eyes as they bored into mine, eyes that questioned our relationship and its purpose. "How can I help you?" I asked, looking at the slowly emerging grimace on his face as he rubbed his shins.

There was an awkward silence as he waited for the translation of my question, and then he simply said, "My legs hurt."

I looked down and noticed his shoes. They were too small, with the fronts cut out to make way for his big toes, which were ready to go out and explore the world. He didn't complain, however, because he was okay with what he had. I sat before a young boy who felt no shame in wearing shoes too small, his toes bursting through the tips, and thought how vain we are when we look in the mirror and see that our pants are a little tight or that the dress doesn't fit that well anymore. We take them off, put them aside, and maybe pass them on to Goodwill. The boy demonstrated true acceptance of what he had been given, no questions asked—no remorse, no embarrassment, and no asking for something better. He had what he had—what God had placed in his life—and he took on the task, wore his shoes, and moved forward, not wanting more. While the shoes didn't fit, they fit just fine as far as the boy was concerned. This is precisely what our God wants: we may not think that we fit the task given to us, but *He* does. The shoes always fit if we want them to. They may bring a little discomfort, but maybe there's a reason for it, and if we look hard enough and listen closely enough, we'll understand His commands.

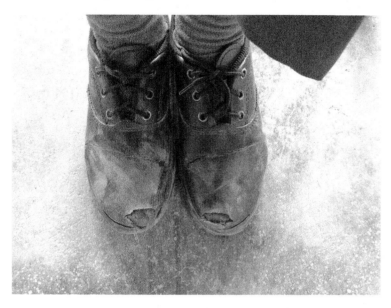

I noticed the girl right away. She was sitting in a row of children, but she wasn't really all there. Her eyes were distant, her affect depressed, and her face showed the picture of a difficult life. As I examined children one after another, I wondered what the odds were that she would come to me. I counted the children sitting in the row and watched the other doctors and nurses who were examining children, still wondering if she would be my next patient. She was.

"How are you feeling?" I asked, looking at her drawn face. She didn't reply.

I tried again. "Does anything hurt?"

The answer I received was one I was hoping not to hear. For some reason it was clear why she looked the way she did. Her wide eyes gave some of it away, and her affect confirmed it. She hadn't eaten dinner the night before and also hadn't eaten lunch. By the afternoon, she'd had only a small glass of milk because her family had no food. She lived with her mother, her older brother, and her grandmother. Her father had traveled to New Delhi to find work so he could send them money. He was a farmer, but his land had been taken away by the government in order to erect a building. India is a large, densely populated country, and individuals get lost and used there just like anywhere else. When I asked "Does anything hurt," she had no answer because, after a certain point in time without food, it really *doesn't* hurt anymore. She was one of the community children we saw after we had examined all of our One Child Matters sponsored children, and I wondered how many more like her there were.

I sat back and thought for a minute just what all this meant. We've all asked this question before of God: Why do you let things like this happen? I, for one, have never gotten a complete or satisfactory answer. We were on our third day of clinics, and I had many questions for God queued up and waiting for answers. What I do know is that when I asked the question, "Where does it hurt," I found myself answering my own question: "My heart hurts."

You would think we could give her money to buy food, or even give her some of our own food, but there's danger in doing that. Being singled out as a "have" in a community that is impoverished brings animosity and jealously. We might have put the girl and her family in great harm, so the best we could do was explore ways to feed the *whole* community, and that wouldn't be an easy task. I asked if I could take her picture, and she said yes. I tried to show it to her, but she looked away, although I'm not sure why. She went on her way with some prayer and vitamins, and as I watched her leave our makeshift medical clinic, my heart sank. We come to serve, and these are the moments when I ask the hard questions of God, waiting for an answer. It seems I'm always listening.

I saw another girl, and she was staring at me, so I naturally speculated about her story. I was in an administrative mode— meeting with the school pastor, talking to a missionary from Kentucky, and making notes for the report I eventually would have to write. Others were tending to patients, and I to my paper and pen. But I kept looking at her as she made her way slowly forward in line, and she kept looking at me. I knew there was a story there, a tap on the shoulder that said "Take notice because I have something to tell you." I couldn't resist. Getting up, I pulled her out of line and took her aside. Using an interpreter, I asked a simple question: "Tell me a little about yourself." Without any prompting from me, she did.

She was six years old, living a life that she described as happy. She went to school, loved her family, wanted to be a doctor (I may have pushed her in that direction a little bit), and loved to eat. No complaints. Life was good, with happy days ahead. Go figure. After the day before, this was a breath of fresh air. How wonderful to see the good side of life and an attitude of acceptance for what little is given us. I hugged her, put her back in line, and walked away singing a tune—"Oh, Happy Day." The little girl had indeed been sent to me. She was one of the answers to my many questions to God, and the answer was that "Sometimes things are good. Stay the course."

The smile is what caught my eye, one that was bright, genuine, and confident—as long as she wore her scarf. I hadn't seen what was below the scarf, but thought it unusual for a young girl to be wearing one. There had to be a reason why it was there, and the bald patches on her head told it all.

I examined her as she walked towards me. She stood barely four feet tall, her clothes were of average quality, and her smile paraded before her. Sitting across from me, she continued to smile until I asked her if it would be okay for me to look at her scalp. She mumbled, and the warm smile turned to a frown, her eyes diverted to the ground as she became noticeably uncomfortable. I looked at her scalp and then scrolled through WebMD, skimming over the details for the type of balding she exhibited. I shut down the tablet and stared straight ahead, pondering the consequences of what I was going to say next. Smiling, I made a diagnosis with an attitude of assurance rather than judgment, but I doubted that it was one she wanted to hear. Indeed, it was probably going to cement her fears. What mattered was that her situation was a worst-case scenario that could play itself out later in life.

Her condition had manifested itself when she was five or six years old. She was now twelve. Her hair fell out in clumps and it had been happening for years, and nothing she had tried on her own had been effective. Her condition was called alopecia areata, which is sometimes reversible with hydrocortisone, but there's no guarantee that the therapy will work. I gave her several tubes of the medication, knowing that because of her baldness she might never marry, be stigmatized and marginalized, or worse yet, she might marry a much older man who cared nothing about her (as in a forced or arranged marriage). The simple truth is that a dysfunctional society makes up rules as it goes along, blindly hurting many because no one is interested in interacting with the genuine person beneath the "what."

I asked her if I could take her picture. This was a sensitive issue, balancing her dignity against telling her story so that others could learn. I struggled with the decision and eventually felt that she would understand. In just a few short minutes we had established a covenant relationship, with her trusting me to do my best to help her.

So what was the lesson in my interaction with the girl? It was this: we are lucky for who we are, for what we have, and for where we live. What we have is better than good, but for many in India, what they have is worse than bad. For this young girl, I speculated on what life would bring. I hoped it would at least bring some measure of good since her smile deserved nothing less.

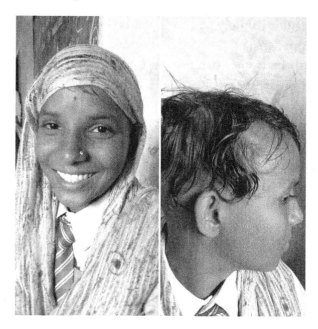

After day six, we'd seen 1,460 patients in four projects, ninety-nine percent of them children. Interestingly enough, the stay seemed far too short. Few of us were anxious to leave the children. Yes, we were eager to return to our families, our homes, and our lives that are so different than what we saw in India, but it was the time we spent with the children that gave us the drive to make their lives better by getting them healthy enough and strong enough to get up in the morning and face their day of poverty. Were we successful? In my book *Covenant Medicine: Being Present When Present*, I write about the four actions that need to be taken when we establish a relationship with our patients: action (how will we change and improve our relationship with our patients); listening (listening to our patients silently); intentionality (focusing on the patient purposefully and willingly); and commitment (treating patients with dignity). Simply put, we are to be "present when present." I'm happy to say that we did all of these things in India. As I watched the twenty-two members of the team performing all four of these aspects of caring, I was in awe at their unselfish giving of themselves. As for the children, I was wonderfully awed at how they came to us. We could speak each other's language courageously, openly, and with trust that is only seen when an unspoken covenant relationship is established.

One of the best known stories in the New Testament is the parable of the Good Samaritan. While two men, a priest and a Levite, passed up a man who had been assaulted and beaten on the road to Jericho, the Samaritan stopped and tended to the man's wounds, pouring oil and wine on them. He then put the man, who had been left for dead, on his donkey and took him to the local inn and paid for the man's stay while recovering. Notice that the Good Samaritan didn't just bandage the wounded man and leave. His care of the victim was complete. He spared neither expense nor time in helping the man to recover, and even stopped at the inn after conducting business elsewhere so he could reimburse the innkeeper for any additional expenses. He had action, focus, intention, and commitment, and he also provided sustainable care to make sure that the man could resume his normal life.

It's a beautiful story. This is not to pat myself or my team on the back and make a pretense at being holier than thou, but it is what is required if we are going to help those in the third world, for they are, in reality, no different than the victim by the side of the road to Jericho. They have been beaten down by life, and people pass them by daily, unwilling to help. They are in plain view, but the senses of those around people who are hurting badly have been numbed. What is necessary is that we notice them and stop and enter into covenant. It is what Christ did for us and, in turn, what we are expected to do for others.

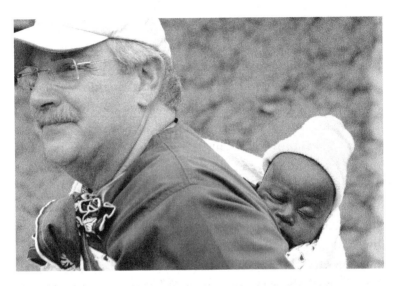

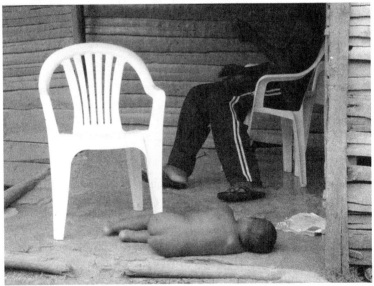

Chapter Thirty-six

Go Therefore
Unto the Whole World

There will be more trips until the day when God tells me that He has other plans for me. The paradox is that, as mentioned earlier, I'm never quite ready for such a radical and swift cultural change when I jump to far-off locations, and yet I am energized once I arrive in a third-world country and begin to interact, along with my team, with the people who come to us for help. Whether I am met with smiles or desperation, I get excited about the possibility of helping our patients, especially the children. There is something in the way the poor and needy look into my face and the faces of my team that immediately overcomes any culture shock and moves us in the direction of establishing covenant relationships.

What will also continue are those questions queued up and awaiting answers from God. As can be seen in the chapters of this book, there are many things I don't understand, such as when God says no to certain individuals or non-sponsored children. I have theories, many of which I've described in the preceding pages, but there are times when I encounter someone who shouldn't have to suffer—someone who will almost certainly face a lifetime of hardship that might be prevented if advanced treatment and facilities were available—and that's when the questions come again. I guess they might all be collected under the umbrella of "Why isn't there justice in these situations, especially after so much prayer?" And yet there is much reflection as I cruise at 38,000 feet, returning from halfway around the world. So I wonder . . .

Justice. It's what we all want, of course. Jesus addressed the issue in an extended parable, which I think appropriate to quote in its fullness.

> Then Jesus told his disciples a parable to show them that they should always pray and not give up. He said: "In a certain town there was a judge who neither feared God nor cared what people thought. And there was a widow in that town who kept coming to him with the plea, 'Grant me justice against my adversary.'" For some time he refused. But finally he said to himself, "Even though I don't fear God or care what people think, yet because this widow keeps bothering me, I will see that she gets justice, so that she won't eventually come and attack me!" And the Lord said, "Listen to what the unjust judge says. And will not God bring about justice for his chosen ones, who cry out to him day and night? Will he keep putting them off? I tell you, he will see that they get justice, and quickly. However, when the Son of Man comes, will he find faith on the earth?" (Luke 18:1-8/NIV)

Jesus exhorts us to be persistent in prayer and never give up, promising that justice will eventually—and always—be dispensed, but He also adds that sometimes justice is delayed by the Father. And so there it is. Justice is sometimes postponed even though it is promised for all in the long run. The passage, therefore, is comforting and troubling at the same time, validating my own angst that not everything happens according to my timetable or according to my wishes. As Pastor Stanley told me so many years ago when I'd been called out to help Baby Nicole, it's all about faith. I didn't think Nicole stood a chance, but she pulled through. I hope and pray that this is the case for many patients we treat, not knowing what their ultimate fate will be.

If we are to take Jesus at His word—and that is always advisable, is it not—we must therefore live with some degree of uncertainty, leaving the details in His hands while keeping faith alive until the day He returns. But how do we live with the questions that keep rising to the surface, the ones that keep surfacing from the depths of our thoughts? I have come to believe that our calling is to focus on continuing the work— persistence, faith, prayer, and good works—and maybe this is an answer in itself. We are told to comfort the sick, feed the hungry, clothe the naked, and visit the prisoner. When we do these things, Jesus said, we do them to Him. At the end of the day, I choose to trust that God, a just judge, will honor my persistence in laboring in His fields. If an unjust judge grants rights, how much more will the one who is justice personified see that all accounts are one day reconciled and balanced? In the meantime, my job is to stay vigilant and keep to my tasks.

It all goes back to the day when, at age eleven, I saw the crowd of Somali tribesmen standing idly by a warrior who had been mauled by a lion. I jumped from the Land Rover because I had to do something. For me, just watching wasn't an option. I'm still doing that today, and sometimes all I receive, as then, is the touch of a hand and a smile. The dying Somali said, "Thank you," and for me and my patients, that is a form of justice. The problem hasn't been ignored, and God has weighed in through His servants. "I see you," he says, "and I love you. You are never forgotten."

And maybe there's an even bigger issue when it comes to finding answers and dealing with injustice. Perhaps another answer to my ongoing question of "Why?" is that we are expected to enter into a larger covenant relationship with the many people—even entire countries—of the world. Are we, as individuals and national entities, going to be present to our brothers and sisters across the globe? Are we going to truly listen non-judgmentally to what they are saying? Are we going to respond with meaningful, compassionate action? Are we going to one day beat our swords into ploughshares as we tend to the sick, the hungry, and the prisoner? While we are waiting for God to dispense His justice, perhaps He, too, is waiting on us to be the agents of that justice. Whatever His master plan is, we are most assuredly a part of it. At a time when the world is at a tipping point, with numerous crises threatening mankind's survival, we can stand idly by and do nothing, or we can become responsible stewards of the earth and partners with our brothers and sisters who inhabit it with us. The choice is ours. Turning my question upside down, maybe it's not God saying, "No." Maybe it is we are not listening to His words and acting on them. Puzzled, we stare at injustice, but maybe it is staring back at us, waiting for a collective response, putting an end to pain and unfairness in His name

To do these things is perhaps risky business, the proverbial fool's errand in a world so fraught with indifference, self-absorption, and materialism. Jesus showed us that the way of path of love and peace was the true and right path. It was the nonviolent way of the cross, on which Jesus gave the utmost in heroic covenant care. For me, it is the only way ahead, walking with Him to the best of my ability. I will continue to heal the sick and wounded in His name, always with humility since He was the one who chose me from the time I was a small child living abroad with my father.

Medical Mercy as an organization is coming to an end. I founded "Covenant Medicine" when I wrote the book "Covenant Medicine: Being Present when Present" and it has lead to a new medical ministry called "Covenant Medicine Outreach". The mission and vision is the same as it was for Medical Mercy, but we will be serving all who come to us, not just sponsored children and putting in place sustainable care for villages and more, in collaboration with local healthcare providers and health ministries. We will be present when present when all patients come to us for help.

The journey continues.

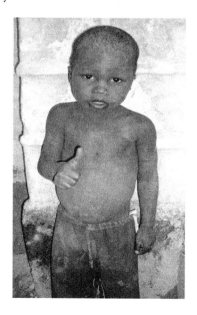

CPSIA information can be obtained
at www.ICGtesting.com
Printed in the USA
FSOW03n1516230816
24061FS